"In *'Dear Institute . . .'*, Himanshu Agraw collective of analysts-in-formation who offer courageous accounts of their experience the structure of the book and the individual contributions integrate past and present, internal and external, individual and institutional points of view. A short history of the contributor's institute is shared at the beginning of each piece. The institute's current contributions to, and sometimes interferences with, the formation of a developing analyst are portrayed. The sum of the book's parts inspires a serious look at the ingredients of training, formal and informal, that contribute to the formation of curious, creative, rigorous graduates. This book is a must-read for analysts involved in psychoanalytic training and an enticing roadmap for those who consider becoming a psychoanalyst."

**Harriet Wolfe**, *MD, President,*
*International Psychoanalytical Association*

" *'Dear Institute . . .'* is a wonderful gift to the entire international psychoanalytic community and beyond. The letters collected here from 40 analysts-in-formation from almost all regions of the world continue an intergenerational dialog that began with 42 letters from older psychoanalysts to the younger generation in *Dear Candidate* and is now proving extraordinarily fruitful. Each letter is fascinating in its very personal description of the changing experiences, the struggle with hopes and wishes but also inner doubts and external obstacles in psychoanalytic training, such as problems with the time available, the costs of training or institutional conflicts. The opportunity to talk emerges as groundbreaking for all these questions: both with older psychoanalysts and within the younger generation, at the local Institute and internationally within the International Psychoanalytical Studies Organization (IPSO). Critical and grateful comments are in a creative interplay. The diverse suggestions in this partly poetic book are essential for the future of psychoanalysis in a changing world. My thanks to all contributors!"

**Dr. med. Heribert Blass**, *President-elect,*
*International Psychoanalytic Association*

"More than an answer, *'Dear Institute . . .'* establishes a rich and truthful dialog with all those interested in psychoanalysis.

"Following the success of *Dear Candidate*, this book presents a cartography of psychoanalytic training around the world. Here, we find love, doubts, ideals, passions, gratitude and creativity; in short, a human and dreamy perspective on the future of psychoanalysis and a testimony to psychoanalytic formations.

"With its unique wealth of images, *'Dear Institute . . .'* offers the reader dreams and distant lands, desire and thirst for knowledge, the past and the search for the unknown.

"Happy reading!"

**Thércio Andreatta Brasil,** *President of the*
*Organization of Latin American Candidates*

"The process of becoming a psychoanalyst evolves throughout our professional lives, but a critical phase of that journey is the deeply personal and immersive experience of training and education in our psychoanalytic institutes and centers. Motivated by his own self-reflection, courage, curiosity, creativity, and humor, Himanshu Agrawal, an advanced candidate at the Minnesota Psychoanalytic Institute, invited 40 candidates/analysts-in-formation from 30 countries to write about their experiences in the form of a letter to their institutes. The result is the revelatory edited volume, 'Dear Institute . . .', comprising intimate and illuminating narratives of the lived experiences of thoughtful, insightful individuals in psychoanalytic training programs around the world. 'Dear Institute . . .' is the international, intergenerational dialogic partner of *Dear Candidate,* a seminal volume of letters edited by Fred Busch and written by senior analysts who share their reflections with candidates. Each volume stands alone, but together, they provide complementary windows into the challenges faced by analysts at different stages of formation and into the complexities and contradictions of the institutional context of their professional lives. Wherever you locate yourself along the spectrum of analyst-in-formation, or if you are simply curious about contemporary psychoanalytic training and education, you will find *'Dear Institute . . .'* richly rewarding."

**Wendy Jacobson**, *MD, Head, Department of Psychoanalytic Education, American Psychoanalytic Association*

"Every future analyst has a home, a real "emotional residence" for his nascent Professional Self: that is, his Training Institute. And he has his own "analytic family" in which he grows both scientifically and humanly, reliving at a deep level the complex path of intergenerational transmission of skills.

"The achievement of technical maturity and work autonomy will never cause him to lose his deep inner connection with this original training environment.

"Those interested in knowing how a psychoanalyst is really trained should read this very book: they will then be able to understand "from the inside," from the authentic testimony of its protagonists, the challenging human journey that leads to the practice of this "impossible," fascinating, adventurous profession."

**Stefano Bolognini**, *MD, former President, International Psychoanalytic Association*

"This volume containing thirty-nine letters from analysts in training from different parts of the world is a crucial contribution to all of us who share a passion for the transmission of psychoanalysis.

"Its diversity in terms of geography, time zones, languages and culture is a remarkable testimony of the commitment to the analytic method and its practice around the world at difficult times following the pandemic, climate tragedy and wars.

"The sincerity and honesty with which the writers of the letters share with us the positive and negative aspects of each of their formative experiences are really moving.

"Together with *Dear Candidate*, the book that inspired the editor to compile these letters, they produce an effect of beauty similar to what in music is called counterpoint: the "art of combining, according to certain rules, two or more different melodies."

"This book is a powerful contribution not only for those interested in psychoanalytic education but even more important for the sustenance of our discipline."

**Virginia Ungar**, *MD, former President,*
*International Psychoanalytic Association*

"'*Dear Institute* . . .' is a remarkable book inspired by *Dear Candidate*, edited by Fred Busch, with letters from 42 analysts from all over the world about their own personal and analytic experience. '*Dear Institute* . . .' is written by 39 analysts in training from 29 countries across the world, candidly sharing their own experiences with their Institutes in the long process of becoming an analyst. As I was reading this moving and unique book, I relived my own analytic journey and had the double feeling of revisiting my past and listening to the thoughts and feelings of our younger colleagues. I strongly recommend this outstanding book that constitute, by its own merits or jointly with its inspiring one, a lively witness of the vitality and creative dialogue among minds, ideas, experiences and generations that are involved in the endless work of building psychoanalysis."

**Prof. Dr. Cláudio Laks Eizirik**, *MD, PhD training analyst,*
*Porto Alegre Psychoanalytic Society and former President,*
*International Psychoanalytic Association*

"This book is 'a must to read'! Reading the vast collection of letters written by analysts in training from all over the world will not only immerse you in the memories of your own training, but it will, above all, introduce you to the richness and variety of what transmission of psychoanalysis today represents.

"Each letter in itself is written with deep thoughtfulness, honesty, and emotion and relates an idiosyncratic experience that is both personal and collective of what the complex path "of becoming an analyst" represents. The reader will have the chance to discover the variety of the different training models around the IPA community, with its strengths and vulnerabilities to be taken into consideration.

"This book will be of great interest not only for the next generation of candidates but also for the training analysts, institutes, and whole members of IPA, as becoming an analyst is a lifelong process, an unending Odyssey!"

**Dr. Katy Bogliatto**, *MD, IPA Vice-President elect*

# "Dear Institute . . ."

This book is a collection of commentaries by 40 psychoanalysts-in-training spanning across 29 different countries, shedding light on the state of contemporary psychoanalysis – its training, practice and relevance.

The perception and landscape of typical psychoanalysis, the typical psychoanalyst and the typical psychoanalytic trainee have witnessed a tectonic shift since Dr. Sigmund Freud first introduced this technique over a hundred years ago. This book challenges and inspires us to think, at all levels, about reimagining how psychoanalysis should be taught in the 21st century. Inspired by Fred Busch's *Dear Candidate* (Routledge, 2021), chapters are written in the style of personal letters from candidates to their faculty and institutes. Each contributor shares a piece of their mind – and their heart – about the trials and tribulations of the process of psychoanalytic training – what they cherished, what they loathed, why they spoke up and why they dropped out.

This book is an important read for both prospective candidates as well as veteran psychoanalysts and institutional leaders.

**Himanshu Agrawal** hails from New Delhi, India, and is currently an associate professor of psychiatry and behavioral medicine at the Medical College of Wisconsin, Milwaukee (USA). He is a psychoanalyst-in-training at the Minnesota Psychoanalytic Institute (USA).

# "Dear Institute . . ."
## Candid Commentaries from Candidates in Psychoanalytic Training

**Edited by Himanshu Agrawal**

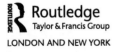 Routledge
Taylor & Francis Group

LONDON AND NEW YORK

Designed cover image: © Getty Images

First published 2025
by Routledge
4 Park Square, Milton Park, Abingdon, Oxon OX14 4RN

and by Routledge
605 Third Avenue, New York, NY 10158

*Routledge is an imprint of the Taylor & Francis Group, an informa business*

© 2025 selection and editorial matter, Himanshu Agrawal; individual chapters, the contributors

The right of Himanshu Agrawal to be identified as the author of the editorial material, and of the authors for their individual chapters, has been asserted in accordance with sections 77 and 78 of the Copyright, Designs and Patents Act 1988.

*British Library Cataloguing-in-Publication Data*
A catalogue record for this book is available from the British Library

ISBN: 978-1-032-73677-8 (hbk)
ISBN: 978-1-032-73675-4 (pbk)
ISBN: 978-1-003-46540-9 (ebk)

DOI: 10.4324/9781003465409

Typeset in Optima
by Apex Covantage, LLC

"Dedicated to my wife Sarah and all the other unsung heroes in the lives of psychoanalytic trainees."

# Contents

# Contributors

**Antonella Trotta-Johnson**

Antonella Trotta-Johnson is a Senior Lecturer in Clinical Psychology at the University of Essex (United Kingdom) and a member of the British Psychoanalytical Society.

**Ashis Roy**

Ashis Roy, PhD and Psychoanalyst, has taught and practiced Psychoanalysis in New Delhi, India. His interest is clinical and cultural psychoanalysis in India and in different South Asian contexts.

**Brigitte Dodge-Johner**

Brigitte Dodge-Johner from Switzerland is a psychotherapist and a member of the Swiss Psychoanalytical Sssociation. She works in her own practice in Lausanne and is an active member of the psychoanalytical institute there.

**Carla Pînzaru**

Carla Pînzaru works in private practice in Bucharest, Romania, and is a psychotherapist trained in psychoanalytic psychotherapy for children, adolescents and adults at Fundaţia Generaţia. She is psychoanalyst-in-training at the Romanian Society of Psychoanalysis.

**Cecilia Caruana**

Cecilia Caruana works in her private practice in Ibiza, Spain. She belongs to the Psychoanalytic Institute of Madrid (APM). She's interested in the analysis and exploration of the human mind from a dynamic point of view in order to help her patients develop a fuller psychic life.

**Chang Jeung Park**

Chang Jeung Park, MD, is a psychiatrist in South Korea and currently runs a private psychiatric clinic as well as a psychoanalytic psychotherapy clinic in Seoul. He is currently pursuing psychoanalyst training at the Korean Institute for Psychoanalysis (KIPSA) and is a candidate representative.

### Cynthia (Cindi) Palman

Cynthia (Cindi) Palman, MD, is a psychiatrist and psychoanalyst. Originally from New York, she now lives and works in Portland and Eugene, Oregon. She is a faculty member of the Oregon Psychoanalytic Institute.

### Erika Lepiavka

Erika Lepiavka is a licensed clinical psychologist and psychotherapist training and working in Mexico City at the Sociedad Psicoanalítica de México. She is dedicated to her private practice and to leading the universe of opportunities that IPSO encompasses as the President of IPSO. Her background as a field psychologist among Mexican marginalized populations and her passion for history and for the study of the present times give her, as a psychoanalyst-in-training, a firm conviction that it is also context that shapes the psyche. She was the IPSO Chair for the 27th IPA Congress, Landscapes of the Mind, from Desert to Fire in Cartagena.

### Eva Christina Tillberg

Eva Christina Tillberg is a licensed child and adolescent psychotherapist and a supervisor and university teacher in psychotherapy. She is based in Stockholm, Sweden, working in a full-time private practice. The training at the Swedish Psychoanalytical Institute follows the requirements of IPA according to the Eitingon model.

### Fred Busch

Fred Busch is a training and supervising analyst at the Boston Psychoanalytic Society and Institute. Dr. Busch has published over 80 articles in psychoanalytic literature and three books, primarily on the method and theory of treatment. His work has been translated into 11 languages, and he has been invited to present over 180 papers and clinical workshops nationally and internationally. In 2020, he edited the book *Dear Candidate: Analysts from around the World Offer Personal Reflections on Psychoanalytic Training, Education, and the Profession*.

### Gabriel Rivera Constanzo

Gabriel Rivera Constanzo is a psychologist and psychoanalyst-in-training at the Chilean Psychoanalytic Association (APCh). He is currently vice president of the Organization of Candidates of Latin America (OCAL) and an invited member of the Commission on Training and Transmission of Psychoanalysis of the Federation of Psychoanalysis of Latin America (FEPAL).

### Gagandeep Kaur Makkar

Gagandeep Kaur Makkar hails from India. She is a Clinical Psychologist and currently working as a Student Counsellor at the Indian Institute of Technology Bhubaneswar. Her training in Psychoanalysis is from the Indian Psychoanalytical Society.

## Hildegarde Kochman

Hildegarde Kochman was born in Panama City, Panama. She is a psychologist and family therapist in private practice and an analyst in training from the institute of the Panamanian Association of Psychoanalysis.

## Himanshu Agrawal

Himanshu Agrawal originally hails from New Delhi, India. He is the first candidate at the Minnesota Psychoanalytic Institute (USA) to complete the majority of his psychoanalytic training remotely. He is an associate professor of psychiatry and behavioral medicine at the Medical College of Wisconsin, Milwaukee (USA) where he has an outpatient practice, teaches medical trainees and conducts research.

## Huner Aydin

Huner Aydin is a psychiatrist and psychoanalyst, and she is a member of the Istanbul Psychoanalytical Association, working privately in Istanbul/ Turkey.

## I-Ning Yeh

I-Ning Yeh has successfully fulfilled the educational and professional requirements to qualify for the practice of psychoanalysis and accordingly was admitted in June 2023 as a Direct Member of the International Psychoanalytical Association. She is also currently a consultant geriatric psychiatrist at St. Joseph Hospital, Kaohsiung (Taiwan).

## Jakub Kuchař

Jakub Kuchař, based in Prague, Czech Republic, serves as a faculty member at the Faculty of Arts, Charles University in Prague. He is also a psychoanalyst-in-training at the Czech Psychoanalytic Society and the co-founder of the Czech online journal *Psychoanalyza dnes*.

## Leticia Aydos

Leticia is an analyst-in-training with the Australian Psychoanalytic Society. She is engaged in adult and child and adolescent training, integrated. She is an experienced psychiatrist consulting in private practice in Sydney. Leticia is originally from the south of Brazil, where her interest in psychoanalysis was also born and nurtured by the strong local analytic tradition. During training, Leticia is experiencing multiculturalism and psychoanalysis, making use of supervision with an analyst from Brazil (with APAS' blessing!) and, therefore, witnessing firsthand the strong analytic consistency across continents, cultures and languages.

## Liliana Correia de Castro

Liliana Correia de Castro is currently a psychoanalytic candidate at the Portuguese Society of Psychoanalysis. She is a consultant psychiatrist working in the public health system in OPorto and an invited auxiliary professor of Psychiatry at OPorto University.

### Liza M. Zachrisson

Liza M. Zachrisson is a clinical psychologist and psychoanalyst training at the Instituto Latinoamericano de Psychoanalysis (ILAP), working in private practice in Guatemala City. She is a co-founder of *Lúdica* (a virtual magazine and academic space for the transmission of psychoanalytic ideas) and former university professor and clinical supervisor at various universities in Guatemala.

### Marìa Florencia Biotti

Psychologist, psychotherapist of children and adolescents. Analyst Member of Buenos Aires Psychoanalytic Association (APdeBA) since 2022. She has been Vice President of the Latin American at IPSO (July 2019–July 2023). Currently, she is an assistant teacher in the APdeBA Master "Psychoanalysis Family and Couple" in the subject "Vinculo fraterno" and a member of the Family and Couple Committee (IPA).

### Maria Lival-Juusela

Maria Lival-Juusela is a psychologist and recently graduated psychoanalyst from the Finnish Psychoanalytical Society. She is also a literary researcher with a PhD in the female Bildungsroman. She works in private practice in Helsinki, Finland.

### Michelle van den Engh

Michelle van den Engh, MD, is originally from Switzerland and transited through Australia, the US, and back to Switzerland before landing in Canada. She is a clinical associate professor at the University of British Columbia Department of Psychiatry and a recent graduate from the Western Canada Psychoanalytic Society and Institute.

### Mirella de Picciotto

Mirella de Picciotto is a clinical psychologist, family therapist, psychosomatician, psychoanalyst and a member of the Paris Psychoanalytical Society and the Psychosomatics School of Paris. She currently works in Paris in both private practice and public institutions with adults and families.

### Muriel Gayet

Muriel Gayet is a psychologist working in private practice in Paris, France. She is a psychoanalyst-in-training at the Société Psychanalytique de Recherche et de Formation (Psychoanalytic Society for Research and Training).

### Naftally Israeli

Naftally Israeli is a clinical psychologist from Jerusalem, Israel. For the last 16 years, he has worked in the Psychological Services of the Hebrew University (in Jerusalem) and works today in private practice. He is a candidate for the Israeli Psychoanalytic Society. His book *Emotional Language* (in Hebrew), based on his PhD thesis, was published in 2019. He writes for Israeli children in a magazine called *Einayim* ("eyes" in Hebrew), and as a therapist who also works with children, he is deeply concerned about the effect of war on children.

### Nancy Pei-Ling Yu

Nancy Pei-Ling Yu is a psychiatrist and psychoanalyst. She received her training from the Taiwan Study Group and is currently qualified as an IPA direct member. She has a private practice in Taipei, Taiwan.

### Naoe Okamura

Naoe Okamura, MD, PhD, is a psychiatrist in Tokyo, Japan. She is currently a candidate at the Training Institute of Japan Psychoanalytic Society (JPS) and serves as an IPSO Representative member of the IPA Communications Committee.

### Natacha Julia Delgado

Natacha Julia Delgado is a graduated member of the Argentine Psychoanalytic Association. She holds a degree in Psychology and Translation. She has translated numerous articles, and since the beginning of her training, she has participated in different committees at the Asociación Psicoanalítica Argentina. She is also a member of the IPA Publications Committee. She works in private practice in clinical psychoanalysis in Buenos Aires.

### Nathalie Bissonnette

Nathalie Bissonnette is from St-Bruno near Montreal, Quebec, in Canada. She is a former military officer who decided to pursue a dream. She is now a psychologist in private practice and a psychoanalyst-in-training at the Institut de psychanalyse de Montréal.

### Nick Flier

Nick Flier is a psychoanalytic psychotherapist residing in Stillwater, Minnesota (USA). He served as the president of the Minnesota Psychoanalytic Society from 2022 to 2024.

### Nicolle Zapien

Dr Nicolle Zapien, PhD, is an advanced candidate at the Psychoanalytic Institute of Northern California (PINC) in San Francisco, California, in private practice. She serves on the ethics committee and chairs the visiting scholar committee at PINC.

### Rafael Mondrzak

MD Rafael Mondrzak hails from Porto Alegre, RS, Brazil, and is currently an associate professor at CELG (Luis Guedes Center Study) of Porto Alegre. He is a Psychoanalyst from the Porto Alegre Psychoanalytical Society (SPPA) and also a Member of the IPA Publication Committee (2021–2024).

### Rolands Ivanovs

Rolands Ivanovs, MD, PhD, is a psychiatrist, medical psychotherapist and psychoanalyst-in-training at the Estonian-Latvian Psychoanalytical Society. He is involved in the Training of Psychotherapy residents at the Riga Stradins University and the University of Latvia and works at his private practice in Riga, Latvia.

### Samuel Lannadère

Samuel Lannadère received a Master's degree in clinical psychology from the University of Paris Diderotis. Samuel is a psychologist with a practice in Paris, France.

### Sebastian Thrul

Sebastian Thrul is a senior psychiatrist at Psychiatrie Baselland in Switzerland, where he runs clinics for adult ADHD and gender issues. He is a psychoanalyst-in-training with the German Psychoanalytical Society (DPG) at the Institut für Psychoanalyse und Psychotherapie Freiburg.

### Siobhán Carter-Brown

Siobhán Carter-Brown graduated as a Psychoanalyst with the South African Psychoanalytic Association in 2022, complementing 16 years of experience in private practice in Johannesburg. Having undertaken various leadership roles in the South African psychoanalytic community, she is dedicated to applying psychoanalysis in a pertinent and meaningful manner in South Africa.

### Susana Maldonado Ponce

Susana Maldonado Ponce is a Mexican psychologist with a Master's degree in Psychoanalytic Research at AMPIEP and is currently an analyst-in-training at AMPIEP. She is the current IPSO's Vice President for Latin America and works in private psychoanalytic practice with children, adolescents and adults. She has participated in and presented papers at national and international congresses organized by AMPIEP, IPSO, OCAL and FEPAL.

**Valentina Palvarini**

Valentina Palvarini is a psychologist with an MA in Infant and Young Observation (Tavistock method) and is a psychoanalyst-in-training at the Training Institute of the Italian Psychoanalytic Society. She lives and works in
Padova (Italy), collaborates with the University of Padova and works with
adults, adolescents and children.

**Ximena Palabé**

Ximena Palabé, born in Uruguay, holds a Bachelor's in Psychology from
the University of the Republic (UdelaR) and a Diploma of Deepening in
Psychotherapy in Health Services Option Psychoanalytic Psychotherapy
from the Graduate School of the School of Medicine of the University of
the Republic (UdelaR). They are an analyst-in-training at the Postgraduate
Institute of Psychoanalysis of the Uruguayan Psychoanalytic Association
(APU).

**Zama Radebe**

Dr. Zama Radebe is from Johannesburg, South Africa, and is currently working as a Clinical Psychologist and a Psychoanalyst in private practice based
in Johannesburg (SA).

# 1 Foreword

*Fred Busch*

Dear Institutes,

Our future is in good hands. After reading these letters from Analysts-in-Formation (AIF),[1] I was left with a feeling of admiration. One cannot help but be impressed with their openness, thoughtfulness, and the clarity of their writing. In general, it was a pleasure to read how they dealt with the personal and professional complexities in being an AIF. Although sometimes it was painful to read about the unempathic comments of senior analysts, in general, this wasn't central in most AIF's experience. Mostly, there was agreement on how important psychoanalytic training was for their professional and personal lives. Finally, I was struck by the maturity of the AIF's letters, especially in their ability to work through ambivalent feelings toward their Institute.

Overall, these AIFs convey important messages about the significance of certain experiences in their training, as well as some problems. I will briefly highlight some trends that stood out for me, but most importantly, these letters deserve careful study as they often serve as a guide to improving psychoanalytic training. Overall, it seemed to me that the AIFs felt that their Institute's training program was "good enough".

Striking was the importance of IPSO for many candidates. This was captured by one AIF who said, "The contact with candidates from other Institutes around the world has brought a multifaceted perspective to training. This has broadened my view of classical and contemporary psychoanalysis and how different training cultures and traditions shape us".[2] Some Institutes view IPSO as so important to the AIF's development that they pay the AIF's dues. At some Institutes, it seems candidates don't seem to know about IPSO and all it has to offer (e.g., the "visiting candidate program" where AIFs can participate in the training of another Institute).

The importance of the group one goes through training with was also mentioned by a number of AIFs. As one AIF stated,

> We also created a great cohort of candidates. We could discuss our perspectives on psychoanalysis with each other and by these discussions

DOI: 10.4324/9781003465409-1

we could consolidate these perspectives more deeply. The important part of these seminars also was, of course, meeting later for a beer and discuss everything regarding our institute informally! At this time, we created bonds that will most likely last till end of our lives.

One Institute encouraged their candidates to bond with their cohort. One AIF who was in an Institute where analysts and AIFs were in seminars together wished for there to be some AIF-only seminars. It was put this way, "I would like a better mix between the "candidates only" ones to acquire the basics and dare ask questions that seem "silly", and the "mixed ones" to deepen and complexify the concepts and thoughts, both clinical and theoretical". My overall impression was that belonging to a group, whether it's the Institute, IPSO, or the cohort one goes through training with, is an important part of the path to becoming a psychoanalyst.[3]

Sometimes, I think Institutes forget how much anxiety there is in applying for psychoanalytic training. Of course, this can be attributed to the AIF's neurosis, but there can also be a reality that should be considered. For example, one Institute had a tradition of having a "meet and greet" event for incoming AIFs, with AIFs already in training and some Faculty members attending, which gave the incoming AIFs the feeling of being part of a group of like-minded individuals. However, one candidate had a different experience.

> I contacted the psychoanalytical Institute I found in my region, full of questions and wondering what the conditions would be. The only thing that came back was a thick envelope. What I understood of the requirements was overwhelming. I felt totally alone and didn't think for a second that anyone on the other side of that envelope might be interested in me . . . Had anyone actually talked to me, reassured me about the expectations and the timeline to get there, it would maybe have been different.

The tendency to interpret the AIF's real difficulties as an unconscious acting out is thankfully hardly mentioned. However, it still exists. One AIF, who was struggling financially, hadn't been paid at the clinic where she worked. After missing a payment to her supervisor, she was confronted by her supervisor, who asked, "If she thought her supervisor deserved to be the one paying for her difficulties". This AIF went on to say,

> Our field is the unconscious, but we have a very real life as well, and it seems to me that we are sometimes quick to only take care of the unconscious or even worse, interpret defensively, or aggressively, in situations where of course there are unconscious fantasies, but reality also exists.

There is, of course, a great deal of anxiety in being an AIF. As one writer put it,

> I sometimes felt and I had to work through the super-egoic function you embody, despite your apparent openness. I could sometimes feel illegitimate and small in front of the weight of the ideal carried by you. I would also have liked to have a more formal return from the supervisors by the end of the supervision, a way to look back together and "wrap up" the work done and the work that was left to be done. But is this too childish a demand?[4]

There is so much more I could say, but I think it best if you hear it from AIFs who have written so openly and honestly about their experiences. I will leave the ending of this Foreword to something written by AIFs that captures the experience of many in these letters.

> Dear Institute, all in all, now that I come to the end of the training, I feel you provided me with "a good enough training" to accompany me on becoming an independently thinking analyst and developing a psychoanalytical identity. It did need for me to have the will to take hold of what you and the Society offers as training tools, at my own pace, and according to my own personal sensibilities and previous personal and professional experiences. I feel I was held in an adaptable envelope with well-defined boundaries and that this appropriate holding device enabled the analyst-to-be (analyste en devenir) that I was six years ago to grow and develop into the analyst I soon hope to be! Going at my own pace also permitted the evolving process of becoming an analyst to unfold with its appropriations, its doubts, its back-and-forth movements, and its elaborating process, in loops that will hopefully bring me to become an always developing and learning analyst.

> I can now say: Thank you.

And from two AIFs writing together:

> In closing we hope that our sharing contributes towards more curious and robust engagements at all levels in our collective. We also hope that we can be part of cultivating an institute that holds space for the candidates and its members to be messy and uncertain, to play with ideas and to dare to explore the stupid. Safety and trust need to be cultivated and protected.

Finally, I would like to thank the creators of this book for inviting me to write this Foreword and for producing this brave and important book. As you know, our book, *Dear Candidate* has led to numerous discussions and webinars across the psychoanalytic world. I hope this book receives the same type of interest and study from Institutes . . . It deserves it.

Fred Busch
Brookline, Massachusetts, USA[5]

## Notes

1  As you will see, some of these letters make a well-thought-out argument, which is not argumentative, for those in analytic training being called AIF rather than "candidates", as we were called during my training.
2  For some AIFs, the book *Dear Candidate* served a similar purpose. After reading these letters, I wish I had named our book, *Dear Analysts-in-Formation*.
3  Most of the AIFs from this group of letter-writers had their training modified during the COVID-19 pandemic, and a few keenly felt the loss of live contact with their cohort and the Institute.
4  This reminded me of two stories from my own time in training. One older graduate analyst told me that in supervision, he felt he never did anything right, and then he graduated. Another analyst told of how his supervisor always told him he was doing fine, and he missed the constructive criticism he knew he needed.
5  One thing that struck me personally was when AIFs described the readings that influenced them, there are no references to North American psychoanalysts, and barely anyone from French authors or the rest of the world. The major influences noted were Klein, Bion, Winnicott, and current authors who follow this tradition.

# 2 Introduction by the editor

*Himanshu Agrawal*

**Common abbreviations used in this book:**

**IPA** International Psychoanalytical Association
**IPSO** International Psychoanalytical Studies Organization
**FEPAL** Federación Psicoanalítica de América Latina
**OCAL** Organization of Candidates of Latin America

## The "developmental history" of this book

I started psychoanalytic training in 2016, and by 2018, I was seriously considering dropping out of training. Since this was no easy decision, I started researching externally and searching internally – and eventually decided to keep going. As luck would have it, I received an opportunity to share my experience through an article I wrote (Agrawal, 2022) in *The American Psychoanalyst* (TAP), the magazine of the American Psychoanalytic Association (APsA). In this article, I described how I was able to work through my idealization of (and ensuing disillusionment with) my psychoanalytic institute. During this journey to explore whether I wished to complete training or throw the towel in, what helped tremendously were the many conversations I had with candidates across the United States of America. These dialogues with fellow candidates ended up being powerful exercises in reality testing and helped me gain crucial perspective. Around the same time, I started reading a book called *Dear Candidate* (Busch, 2020), which contained letters assembled from various graduate psychoanalysts from across the world. Like a timely inoculation, these letters provided words of wisdom and comfort to my dejected soul.

I did not know Dr. Busch too well; however, I was aware that he was kind enough to reply to emails. So, in January 2022, I reached out to him. I thanked him for *Dear Candidates,* and how it served as a soothing balm during difficult times in Psychoanalytic training. I also shared with him – feeling a bit audacious, I must confess – that I had been playing with an idea inspired by his book. The idea was to publish another book with a similar format as *Dear Candidate* except from a different vantage point. The working title

DOI: 10.4324/9781003465409-2

would be *Dear Institute,* and it would essentially be a collection of letters describing what it was like to be a candidate in contemporary times and what this generation of students wished institutes would know and understand. Not only did Dr. Busch reply with words of support, he even agreed to write a foreword for the book!

Next, I reached out to a mentor, who got me in touch with the team at Routledge. They liked the idea and encouraged me to expand my vision from national to global. I reached out to Dr. Harriet Wolfe, who was, at that time, the president of IPA. She introduced me to Charles Baekeland, who was, at that time, the president of IPSO. To my utter disbelief, soon we had 40 candidates, spanning 30 countries and all six inhabitable continents, willing and eager to write their hearts out! For a multitude of reasons and commitments, Charles had to excuse himself from being the co-editor of this book; however, I will forever be indebted to my 'partner' for giving wings to this project.

### From 1915 to 2020

When I thought about how to organize and present the letters in this book, I toggled with many ideas – dividing the letters by prominent themes; presenting them according to the regions of the world they came from; in alphabetical order of the authors, or the countries they hailed from.

Ultimately, I realized that the most befitting organization for a set of messages addressed to organizations dedicated to the importance of developmental years would be to present them according to the years in which these institutes developed.

I have read and re-read these letters in several orders and have found several interesting observations when I read them in chronological order of their 'birth' (defined in this book by the years the institutes were recognized by either the American Psychoanalytic Association or directly by the International Psychological Association). I will contain my observations for a different time, perhaps a different venue, primarily for this reason – I would like you to revel in your own observations and reach your own deductions. Anything else would be ironic in a book dedicated to psychoanalysis!

### "Imperfect English is the language of the international psychoanalytic candidate"

When I set out to edit the first letter I reviewed, I made 128 edits. Charles reminded me of a delightful quote he had heard at an IPA conference—"the language of IPA is bad English!" He encouraged me to discard my neurotic desire to see the letters from an 'America-centric' lens and to embrace the earnest beauty inherent in the nascent forms of the letters. I looked at the same letter with my new lens, and the edits dwindled from 128 to 2. We ask that you consider using a similar lens as you read these letters from all over the world.

Our team has put a lot of care and thought into the editing process. Unless the narrative is distracting or overtly confusing, we have resisted the urge to 'correct' syntax, grammar, and propositions. We have embraced them all – malapropisms, idiosyncratic use of half-remembered idioms, provincial slang, and local spellings. We believe that you will have as much fun churning in your head the pluralities of meaning as you will taking in the clear themes of content.

### The heart of the letters—"share pieces of your mind and your heart!"

The initial communication to all prospective authors contained the following message:

*"We would like for your contribution to this project to take the form of a roughly 3000-word letter to your Institute in which you reflect freely upon your training experience. This can develop many avenues of thought amongst which could be:*

- *what led you to psychoanalytic training,*
- *what your expectations were,*
- *what your personal psychoanalytic experience was/is like,*
- *how your cohort worked together,*
- *your thoughts on seminars, theory, the quality of the teaching,*
- *if institute politics affected training,*
- *your experience with supervisions, etc.*

*We hope that you will share pieces of your mind, and your heart, about the trials and tribulations of the process of psychoanalytic training: what you cherished, what you didn't, why you choose to speak up."*

Additionally, although our team started with the title *"Dear institutes . . .",* somewhere along the process, we started to imagine the Institute as a living, breathing being. In fact, at one point, I started asking the authors to do the same – imagine if their psychoanalytic training institute was a person, what kind of a person would it be? Would it be a benevolent old man in a bow tie and a walking cane? Or would the Institute take the form of a lively, vibrant woman dressed in bright clothes? Perhaps something entirely different – amorphous, ethereal. (And so on and so forth . . .)

You will notice that several of the authors took this suggestion to heart, as inferred by the capitalization of the word 'Institute' when they address it in their letters ('Dear Institute').

As the initial drafts came in, it was clear that the candidates/analysts-in-training had plenty to say. Some letters came in with a brief history of the institute, including important (oft controversial) changes along the way. These pieces of background added important context and seemed to enrich the letter so much that we asked each author to send us a brief report containing graduation requirements and a history of the institute. These have been added to the beginning of each letter, within italics.

Many (but not all) of the first drafts came in as pure love letters. Some of these have remained so, while others took up my request to add a little more 'bite' (admirably, without sounding bitter), as they posit difficult questions and share wishes and desires for the benefit of their successors.

It is my sincerest hope that you will find these letters enjoyable, useful, and perhaps even important – and that you will appreciate the sincerity and vulnerability with which they have been composed.

—Himanshu Agrawal

# 3 A letter to the British Psychoanalytical Society, London, United Kingdom (1913)

*Antonella Trotta-Johnson*

*Founded by Ernest Jones in 1913, the British Psychoanalytical Society includes important figures in the history of psychoanalysis, such as Donald Winnicott, Michael Balint, Wilfred Bion, John Bowlby, Anna Freud, Melanie Klein, Joseph Sandler, Hannah Segal and many more.*

*The World War and Nazi persecutions of Jews during the 1930s and 1940s caused many analysts — Sigmund and Anna Freud included — to flee to London to escape from the horror of the war.*

*Surviving the social, political and psychological turmoil of the two world wars, the British Society grew and evolved to accommodate new members, ideas and attitudes. From the beginning, it has included a significant number of women and also non-doctors and fostered the development of a tradition centred on the psychoanalytic treatment of children.*

*Perhaps one of the most significant events in the history of the Society was the arrival of Melanie Klein to London in 1925, bringing her original theory of internal objects and her pioneering clinical technique. A group of supporters formed around her, who were interested in exploring her ideas around the pregenital phase. When refugee psychoanalysts began arriving in London in the 1930s, tension built up between the Viennese immigrants and Klein's followers, who included Rivière, Rickman, Isaacs and, as students, Winnicott, Bion and Bowlby.*

*After Sigmund Freud's death in 1939, rivalries intensified & two distinct groups had emerged centred around Anna Freud and Melanie Klein. During the years between 1941 and 1944, Controversial Discussions within the British Psychoanalytical Society focused on central scientific questions for psychoanalysis (such as the infant psychic life) as well as about the training programme and, more implicitly, about the future identity of the Society.*

*The atmosphere was heated, and there was a great danger of a division of British Society.*

*The discussions culminated in the formation of the Hampstead Clinic group led by Anna Freud, the Kleinian group and the middle group bringing together object relation theorists and non-aligned people.*

DOI: 10.4324/9781003465409-3

*Over the decades, there have been disagreements and debates, and different approaches to psychoanalytic thoughts and practice have emerged. Nevertheless, despite the difficulties to process the conflicts that emerged during the Controversial Discussions, what has remained constant throughout the years is the British Psychoanalytical Society's role as an active, supportive and flourishing centre of psychoanalytic thought and practice in UK and internationally.*

*The requirements for qualification at the British Psychoanalytical Society are:*

- *Completion of infant observation for one year duration, including attendance of weekly infant observation seminars throughout the first year of training and a final written report about the experience once it is finished.*
- *Evening seminars two or three times a week. These include weekly clinical seminars in small groups and one or two theoretical seminars. In years 1 and 2, the theory seminars are compulsive, then candidates can choose which theory seminars they'd like to attend. A minimum of 52 credits combining lectures and seminars and including all compulsory seminars (attendance at five seminars represents one credit) is required for qualification.*
- *Personal analysis: candidates must have completed at least one year of five times a week analysis with a Training Analyst for the Institute to apply for the training and personal analysis with a Training Analyst must continue throughout the duration of the training.*
- *Two cases under supervision (weekly), one male and one female case. A minimum of two years' clinical work with the first case and one-year clinical work with the second case in 5x weekly analysis is necessary to apply for qualification.*

—

Dear Institute,

It was a Friday evening, about seven years ago, when I attended your Open Evening.

Like the memory of my first day at school, it is still quite vivid. I remember sitting nervously at the back of the Sigmund Freud Lecture Theatre; I was curious and, at the same time, quite doubtful about the idea of starting the training.

Coming from abroad, I have always felt uncertain about the long-term commitment to Psychoanalysis in a foreign country, training in a foreign language, and I was also frightened by having to learn the language of Psychoanalysis, which sounded to me even more alien than English.

At the same time, I was attracted to the idea of being part of the British Psychoanalytical Society with its long international, culturally diverse tradition, which, during the training, I have learnt welcomed many migrants like me, in search of a safe place to be.

*I wasn't personally escaping from the horrors of a World War*, nevertheless, I was looking for a space to learn and grow, as a candidate as well as a young woman.

Several years later, I now feel deeply grateful to have the opportunity to go through and share my own experience of training while I am still fully immersed in it. The word immersed comes to mind while I start writing this commentary. Perhaps because of my visceral attachment to the Mediterranean Sea, the landscape where the seeds of my interest in Psychoanalysis started growing. I wonder whether growing up in the proximity of a Volcano, a giant that nurtures yet that can destroy, has drawn me to become interested in the unconscious aspects of the mind.

It has been a long journey to get to the Institute, with many detours.

I first trained as a Clinical Psychologist in the South of Italy and worked for the National Health Service in psychiatric hospitals with people going through psychotic breakdowns.

Once qualified, I had the opportunity to spend six months in London, something I could not miss. I was planning to return to my country after this short experience . . . but . . . more than 10 years later, I can say that my plans have transformed radically.

This was the beginning of a complex relationship, a relationship that changed my career plan unexpectedly but mainly it has changed my whole life and brought me emotionally closer to Psychoanalysis. As with every relationship, it has not been always smooth.

The first few years in London were quite unsettling; I felt displaced and destabilised, like an alien landing from an island to a new island. I remember 2011 as the year of Riots that happened in London, but also in my own mind.

However, this unsettling time was also extremely rich and transformative.

As a stepping stone, I first approached another Institution, the Tavistock and Portman, and began weekly psychotherapy with an Analyst from the Society. It was during a training course at the Tavistock that I met the person who later became my Training Analyst.

She helped me to recognise my need to become an analytic patient first, and perhaps she was the first person who truly believed that I could become an analyst long before I did.

A few years later, after a preliminary interview with a senior analyst of the Society, I was invited to apply for the training. Alongside my PhD thesis, I wrote my application to the Institute of Psychoanalysis, and the latter was definitely the most challenging writing up for me. It took nine months, as every question opened up new spaces within myself stimulated thoughts and feelings. It was perhaps the first time I could write the narrative of my life at my own pace.

The result was a more than 40 pages long application. I then was invited to attend two interviews of about 1.5 hours each. I felt very anxious of being rejected, not knowing how and what to prepare. I left the interviews thinking 'I will never get through!'. And instead, I made it through . . . my curiosity and excitement grew stronger, as my anxieties.

If I look back, those 40 pages of application were one of the first chapters of my psychoanalytic journey. It has been now six years since I became part of this Institute, and many more chapters of my life as a candidate have definitely been written, others are in the process of being written, others are not fully formed yet in my mind and still trying to make sense of.

The first thing I had to learn from 'day one' of training is how to multitask and juggle work and personal life alongside the commitments required by the training.

Internal and external flexibility has been key to arrange the days, fitting in five times a week personal analysis, at least two evening weekly theoretical and clinical seminars, and over the past three years also two training patients, five times a week, along with two weekly supervisions. It has been a full immersion from the start.

I initially felt intimidated by the 'five times'; however, it is actually the intensity of seeing a patient five times a week that brings an extraordinary depth to the type of analytic work with them. And in my opinion, it is also very much enjoyable most of the time.

Not always . . .

It surprises me, since I have started the training, how time and space have acquired a different dimension. I travel every day from South to North London to work with my training patients, for my own analysis and to attend seminars on the other side of the town. I have estimated around 20 hours of weekly commuting. However, despite this, the years have passed, and I have adjusted to this rhythm; I go through some difficult days when I feel I am stretching my limits, psychic as well as physical, to try to fit 'everything' in. I have felt the exhaustion, and the guilt for leaving everything else behind.

If I go back to the beginning of the training, one of the most relevant experiences in the first year has been the Infant Observation, which is something distinctive of the training at the British Society. The year-long observation of a new-born baby allowed me to think about the mother's and baby's perspectives and the communication between them. It has been a unique experience on how the relationship developed, as one in which the baby could express her needs and the mother responded and contained her distress.

I had very little experience of babies; it was a privilege to be a fly on the wall and just observe in contrast with my daily job as a health professional and academic, where I feel the external and internal pressure to act and come up with treatment plans or make decisions about other people's lives. The experience of the observation made me also think about the infant within myself; it made me reflect on my own early development, the relationship with my mother and I also reflected on the possibility of imagining myself as a mother in the future, something that I have been mostly avoiding thinking about up to that moment.

Alongside the observation of the baby, participating in clinical and theory seminars was another core component of the training that I really enjoyed in the first years. Some seminars are flagship courses and recommended to attend by the end of the training, enriched by the three British traditions, the Contemporary Freudian, Kleinian and Independent, that have found a way to dialogue together creatively in the Society.

And the combinations between evenings and weekend seminars, small and bigger groups' discussion, mixing with other candidates at different stages of the training and from a variety of cultural and professional backgrounds is what makes the learning particularly enriching and diverse. As candidates, we are also encouraged to be part of the vibrant British Psychoanalytic community from the outset. For example, by participating to the scientific meetings, regional colloquiums, English Speaking Conference and contributing to the internal Bulletin.

I have been an active member of the Student Organisation Body of the Institute of Psychoanalysis (SOBIPA), which is a place to voice our opinions on psychoanalytic training standards, support each other throughout the training and represent the candidates' group at a local and international level. Since the second year of training, I have taken on the role IPSO representative in my Institute, which has now become a 'working party' with other candidates, that meets to think together how to foster the international links with other Institutes across the Channel. And it is through IPSO that I have the opportunity to write up this commentary.

By sharing all these experiences with my peer group, I have developed close friendships, some colleagues have become part of my extended family in and out of London, we meet outside the training, and with some it has become a close connection that I hope will last for a lifetime.

Alongside the enthusiasm, involvement, and idealisation of the journey at the initial stage of training, I have noticed that over time I entered a different state of mind and started seeing my experience of training through different lenses.

Surely, but not only, the pandemic has been like a psychological earthquake that has shaken my identity as a candidate, with the necessity to quickly adjust the training experience to these dramatic circumstances.

For almost a year, I have had remote communication with my patients, with my own analyst, supervisors, and progress advisor. Since then, theoretical and clinical seminars as well as the scientific meetings have been happening as regularly as before, but mainly on a virtual space that feels more distant.

Going back to the initial metaphor of the immersion in the water, dear Institute, there have been moments that I have felt like swimming in troubled water, trying to keep my head outside but feeling a strong pull down. Sometimes, being a candidate has amplified my personal insecurities and the sense of uncertainty in my daily life.

One of these moments was when my second training patient dropped out from the analysis, a few months before I could qualify. For some time, I went through a sense of loss and carried an open wound that was difficult to heal.

I have felt angry, responsible, carried a sense of shame for the abrupt departure, having to reapply for permission to the Student Progress Committee, join a waiting list for another patient, and not knowing when this was going to happen; I felt as if I was put in limbo. My personal analysis was the place where I could express my ambivalence towards this stage of training, whilst supervision was a helpful place to learn from this experience.

However, I now believe this was a turning point in my life, not only as candidate, a point where I finally had to negotiate my expectations about the training and let go of the ideal training and the ideal candidate I had in mind, which was far away from reality.

Like on a roller coaster, I have gone through moments of illusion and disillusion, losing motivation but also having the opportunity to opening unknown doors and exploring new territories, developing new friendships, and finding new meaning to the journey I have embarked upon.

And my own analysis, my life outside the Institute, being part of the international IPSO network has been a major source of support to go through troubled waters, and has kept me going.

Perhaps I have entered a new phase, less like a dream either black or white, but can appreciate more the colour nuances of what it is like being in training.

I have doubts and uncertainties about getting closer to the ending of the training and beginning the journey of becoming an analyst, as I had when I sat at the Sigmund Freud Lecture Theatre during the Open Evening.

And a question that I would like to ask myself and perhaps my Analyst, Supervisors, training committee members and Progress Advisor is: *what's next?*

For the future, I hope the Institute could provide more space, in the clinical and theoretical components of the training, to engage together with the new generations of candidates in thinking about ethnicity and culture, to stimulate an ongoing critical reflection and emotional understanding of the interplay between societal and intrapsychic dynamics, and how psychoanalysis could contribute to discussions of these important issues both inside and outside the consulting room.

— Antonella Trotta

# 4   A letter to the Paris Psychoanalytic Institute, France (1915)

*Mirella de Picciotto*

*In France, there are three IPA (International Psychoanalytic Association) societies that have very similar training models but quite different styles, and many non-IPA societies. The Paris Psychoanalytic Institute (IPP) is the training institute of the Societe Psychanalytique de Paris (SPP), which is the first psychoanalytical society created in France (by Freud and Marie Bonaparte in 1915).*

*The IPP does not follow the Eitingon model.*

*The prerequisites to start training are:*

- *At least three years of personal analysis with an IPA member prior to the demand to start training (only the name of the analyst is asked)*
- *Meeting three training members of the Society that will evaluate the readiness of the applicant to start training*

*The training entails:*

- *Two control cases for at least two years, and a minimum of three sessions per week. One supervision is individual, the other one is in a small group (collective supervision). A paper is written by the candidate for each case and addressed to the supervisor.*
- *A free choice of seminars*
- *Meeting with two training analysts at the end of one's training before validation*

—

Dear Institute,

Now that the time has almost come to leave you, I look back on the path I have taken six years ago when I decided to write to you to express my desire to become an analyst and undertake the training you offer.

It has now been five years that I have been traveling the road you set up for candidates to become analysts. My desire to become an analyst had been

DOI: 10.4324/9781003465409-4

long withstanding and dated back to when I was only a teenager. It consistently reaffirmed itself through my personal analysis and my experience as a psychologist and child psychotherapist in public institutions. However, it looked like a huge step to move forward and to put it into action and words. I guess you represented for me such an ideal that I felt illegitimate to want to enter. The transference took place from parental figures, through my analyst, to you "The Institute"! I felt all your eminent figures looking down at me, and your power and narcissistic struggles looked to me like a battle of Titans. It, therefore, took a long way and the elaborations of my personal analysis to make it possible for me to embrace the path to join you. Legitimacy was a major issue, of course: why did I want to become an analyst, what was the best way for me to become one and could I become a "good enough"[1] analyst for my patients? I believed I needed a framework that was at the same time solid and open, and that would enable me to benefit from the transmission of experienced analysts I respected, and you seemed to provide that. I was looking for a listening ear that could enlighten me on my blind spots and that could help me better work with my patients. It was important for me to learn and better understand the working of the mind and that included the emotional aspect of it. Considering the other French psychoanalytical societies, you seemed like the best fit for me.

First and foremost, you are the institute of my analyst's society! However, I did not choose you only because of transference matters. I had had a first analysis with a member of another society, which left me very unsatisfied and since I found my second analysis with an SPP member much more fruitful, I inferred that your training was "better". Moreover, the cohort in training is about 200 candidates, and the society (SPP) comprises about 800 members. I felt that gave room to the possibility to explore different theoretical and clinical viewpoints and work with a large variety of analysts to find and construct my own psychoanalytical identity. I felt you would provide me with the appropriate tools to start my work as an analyst and then continue to learn and elaborate within the Society.

It might look like a semantic preciosity (but as analysts, we do know how important words are), but I do cherish it that you call us neither "candidates" nor "élèves" (pupils) like you used to, but "analyste en formation" which translates as "analyst in training". It displaces the focus off the educational aura, as *psychoanalysis can't be taught* as such; it is first foremost a personal experience, and a transformation and integration of a transmission. Like in English, formation has a double meaning in French; not only does it entail training and putting into shape, but it also contains the idea that when we go through the training, we are to "form" a psychoanalytic identity for ourselves. And this formation is a process, one could say like the one which transforms a caterpillar into a butterfly, each with its own colors and patterns. The difference of course is that the formation of an analyst is a psychic and internal one. But that process takes time, and a different amount of time for each one of us. Like the process of the analysis, the process of the formation of the analyst takes the pace needed by the internal transformations required to become one, and I feel you allow this flexibility of timing that each one needs to achieve it, while still offering a frame that provides a "good enough holding" as Winnicott (1960) would say. Experiencing it felt sometimes puzzling and frightening because of the doubts and uncertainties our work contains, as we are alone in the consulting room with our patients, and at other times so enriching when the analytical process unravels.

I am also grateful to you for having provided me with a structure "malleable enough" that left space not only for my own maturational pace, but also for experiencing and challenging my own desire. The way you structure training entailed for me as a candidate to build my own path according to my interests and affinities. My desire was thus set into motion, and I felt in charge and responsible for carrying it through. I had to work through my ambivalence, confront my idealization of you and work through the de-idealization that necessitated a mourning process. This process echoed the transference one in my personal analysis and made me work through it again.

Dear Institute, I also feel very important and value the fact that you are a "non-reporting" institute and had no meddling with my personal analysis. This barrier protects the intimacy needed for an analytic treatment to be authentic. By preserving the space of personal analysis separate from training, only ensuring that the candidate's analysis has been with an IPA member, I believe you make a good compromise between assuring a minimum security about the personal analysis of the analyst-to-be and the need for intimacy that the analysis itself requires in order for it to be truthful. Furthermore, since the question of the analyst's place in the Society is not a variable of the choice, I felt free to choose the analyst that I felt suited me best.

However, this freedom has its downsides, of course. For example, once I was accepted to the training, a wide choice of seminars and supervising analysts opened up. You strongly suggest some seminars for the training but make nonmandatory. What an horizonless ocean! How could I choose between all these fascinating seminar titles, what was within or beyond my reach, where to start from?

I was lucky enough to work already in clinical institutions with SPP analysts, and thus could discuss my hesitations with them, be guided in some of my choices. Only recently, seeing that this freedom drove some analysts in training to feel lost, did you start bringing more branches to lean on: you now give us a referent with whom we can meet to discuss our training path and the questions or difficulties we come to struggle with. Also, we now meet with you every two years in order for you to better accompany us on our way to validation.

Dear Institute, I must say that I sometimes felt that you were not providing me with enough guidance and that constructing a solid and coherent theoretical baggage was a big responsibility to carry on my own. However, must we not learn to walk autonomously in order to grow, even if it sometimes entails taking some risks and even sometimes falling on the way? As you can see, this training sometimes drew me back in time and brought back child-hood issues. My fellow mates and I sometimes feel you are infantilizing us, and we complain about it, but I think it is part of the process to go through this regression in order to elaborate something of one's own analytic stance and learn to stand alone on one's feet.

Another specificity about the seminars you offer carries great advantages but also downsides. Only one of these seminars is specifically intended for candidates. It is held in a small group (15 participants) with two training ana-lysts. Clinical situations and theoretical texts are worked through over the weekend and informal times are shared. All the other seminars are open and attended both by members and candidates, which I mostly feel is very enrich-ing. It is a great way for us to have access to high quality discussions about both clinical and theoretical matters and to experience different, and some-times confrontational viewpoints. It also helps us develop critical thought and de-idealize analytic thinking. Moreover, I strongly believe that these shared seminars help the transition between being a candidate and becoming a member and fosters the cohesiveness between you and the Society we will later belong to. Having said all of that, dear Institute, in these mixed seminars, I was sometimes overwhelmed by the feeling of lacking so much knowledge and thus not being able to follow the discussion. I must not have been the only one because candidates rarely speak up in these joint seminars! I some-times think that both types of seminars are needed and are complementary; the "candidates only" ones to acquire the basics and dare ask questions that seem "silly", and the "mixed ones" to deepen and complexify the concepts and thoughts, both clinical and theoretical.

As for the supervisions, in order to qualify for the validation of the training, you ask us to complete two supervised cases of analysis three times a week on the couch, for at least two years each. At least one of the analyses has to be a treatment paid by the patient in order for us to experience and analyze matters related to payment, transferentially and countertransferentially. You let us choose our own supervisor, and it was very important for me to choose a benevolent supervisor because my own Superego was already looking over my shoulder with enough roughness! And here again, alongside the indi-vidual supervision for one of our patients, you have created a specificity for our other training case, the "collective supervision". Four of us meet weekly for two hours with one training analyst and we each report the material of our second control case. I found this setting precious because in these col-lective supervisions, we can hear other fellow candidates talk about their own patient with their own personal style. We can then experience alterna-tive sensibilities and ways of hearing the material in its various aspects. We realize how our intervention styles are personal to each one of us and can put these differences to work collectively. Thus, both horizontal and vertical transmission and learning are fostered. Additionally, it was a pleasure for me to join my colleagues every week and share with them our frustrations and satisfactions. I feel it is also a way of fostering long lasting bonds which can even develop into friendships between "supervision brothers and sisters" (if the fraternal rivalries are not too sharp!). This form of "group training" favors a sense of belonging to the group, first the supervision group, then the Society and lastly the IPA. For my part, this aspect of training was very enriching and added the pleasure of developing interpersonal relationships with future colleagues in the Society to the interest of learning and working together.

An important aspect of my training also took place on the side of the classical training curriculum you offer. Participating as a co-therapist in two groups of psychodrama with senior and training analysts taught me a lot. I felt this was a great learning place because I could participate actively to the treatment of the patient and benefit from the group discussions and elaborations after each session. Seeing senior analysts at work not only provided identification grounds but also the comforting experience that even they were sometimes at a (relative) loss and still searching with an open mind how to best understand and help the patient. I came to think that you could encourage all of us candidates to go through this sometimes unsettling but mostly enthralling experience.

Dear Institute, the other space I started working in is closely linked to you. I am referring to the Centre Favreau. You and the Society created the Centre Favreau many years ago, this center where free analytic treatments are given. You allowed some of us to see a patient there in classical analysis as part of our training, while being supervised outside the institution. In my case, having the opportunity to receive my first patient in analysis in this framework helped me in working through my inner resistances to pass "behind the couch". Furthermore, working in the Centre as a candidate, I could benefit from the discussions involving experienced analysts that took place in the bi-monthly clinical meetings and could confront myself with different models of being an analyst with each specific patient.

Last but not least – IPSO! You foster international bonds with candidates from other institutes and pay IPSO for each one of us automatically. I feel it is a clear and strong statement about the need to be open to other psychoanalytic cultures than yours and across borders. As for me, my belonging to IPSO has been a specifically important part of my formation as an analyst. Being Italian, with a multicultural background, both personal and academic, I found in IPSO the perfect field to invest and explore various psychoanalytic cultures that mirrored my international and multicultural personal background. The international activities, Colloquiums, Study Days, pre-congress meetings of the IPA congress and of the FEP (Fédération Européenne de Psychanalyse), enabled me not only to meet candidates from other countries but also to learn about the differences and similarities of our analytic cultures and training models. It offered alternate viewpoints of my own path, put to question my basic assumptions and fostered thought and creativity. It not only made me wish for some changes but also made me appreciate what was already in place. It participated in preventing me from assuming that there is only one truth, one way to think, one way to be an analyst and to practice psychoanalysis. I, for example, realized how, although standing strongly against certain aspects of Lacanian theory, French psychoanalysis, even at the SPP, has been marked by it. IPSO also enabled me to visit BPAS (the Institute of the British Psychoanalytic Society) for two weeks in the framework of the Visiting Candidate Program (VCP). Supervising with British training analysts opened up new perspectives that I brought back with me in France and in my office. Mirroring this experience, as an IPSO representative at the SPP, I welcomed candidates from other societies to my own and helped them organize their VCP program. Dear Institute, I also had the chance to see how you were being watchful and were taking into account what we as candidates had to say about the training you offered us, and that the form of the training was an evolving matter. Seeing you wonder, have doubts, try to find better solutions, adapt according to new challenges – all of this was precious. I could grasp and appreciate that you and the training were not carved into stone, but that you were yourself lively and changing within a solid base. Thanks to IPSO, we built a small group of British and French candidates in order to work together on clinical and theoretical issues, with all the pleasure of meeting one another regularly online and twice a year in person, alternatively in London and in Paris. A whole new set of possibilities to explore and to foster curiosity in our field! I cherish the possibilities that you gave us to carry forth our project, our collective "psychoanalytic baby" one could say! Both the British Institute and you supported us in providing us with a place to meet, and training analysts from each society joined us to discuss our clinical material with great generosity. They also shared aspects of their own psychoanalytical and institutional history. In these times when psychoanalysis is challenged and sometimes carries a negative "reputation" in our hard science and "fast serve-fast fix" societies, I feel it is most important to reach out and keep developing our diversity and overture not only to thrive but also not to risk stiffening on defensive positions that would not only caricature what psychoanalysis is, but also impoverish it.

One last word for a struggle that it sometimes is to endure a psychoanalytic training. I sometimes felt and had to work through the superegoic function you embody, despite your apparent openness. I could sometimes feel illegitimate and small in front of the weight of the Ideal carried by you. I would also have liked to have a more formal return from the supervisors by the end of the supervision, a way to look back together and "wrap up" the work done and the work that was left to be done. But is this too childish a demand? Maybe an important part of the training is that one has to "seize the role", and that partly demands something that is inwardly felt as a transgression. Like going through the transition of teenage years, when one has to separate from one's parents and lean on an internal object, through training, one has to become an analyst by creating an analytical internal object of one's own "against and besides one's masters". Because in the end, in the office and in our chair, we are alone with our patient; what accompanies us are the framework and the different voices that speak within ourselves – our analyst(s), our supervisors,

our seminar directors, our colleagues, our readings . . . and what they fantas-
matically represent!

Dear Institute, all in all, now that I come to the end of the training, I feel you
provided me with "a good enough training" to accompany me on becoming
an independently thinking analyst and developing a psychoanalytical identity. It did need for me to have the will to take hold of what you and the Society offers as training tools, at my own pace and according to my own personal
sensibilities and previous personal and professional experiences. I feel I was
held in an adaptable envelope with well-defined boundaries and that this
appropriate holding device enabled the analyst-to-be (analyste en devenir)
that I was six years ago to grow and develop into the analyst I soon hope to
be! Going at my own pace also permitted the evolving process of becoming an analyst to unfold with its appropriations, its doubts, its back-and-forth
movements and its elaborating process, in loops that will hopefully bring me
to become an always developing and learning analyst.

I can now say: Thank you!

— Mirella de Picciotto

# 5 A letter to the Swiss Society of Psychoanalysis, Switzerland (1919)

*Brigitte Dodge-Johner*

*The Swiss Society of Psychoanalysis (SSPsa) was founded in 1919. It is one of the component societies of IPA and in this context, it is a member of the European Federation of Psychoanalysis (FEP), established in 1966.*

*In agreement with the API, the SSPsa considers that the transmission of psychoanalysis can only take place within an institution. The SSPsa performs this task through regional institutions (cf. Centers).*

*Switzerland follows the French model, but there are two levels of membership, associate and ordinary.*

*To be accepted as a candidate, you need to go to two rounds of interviews with two training analysts each time, with a yearlong wait in-between. Your personal analysis has to be on the way by then.*

*The usual way of training is to pick any seminars at your institute or another institute of the country, following your unconscious choices.*

*To become an associate member, you need*

- *A personal analysis,*
- *A certain amount of clinical and theoretical seminars, and*
- *Two weekly supervised control cases that last for at least two years.*
- *You then present the verbatim of three sessions to a commission who judges on your ability to work analytically with a patient.*
- *When I started, the requirement to become an aM was that one of the two analysis had to be at a four weekly sessions frequency; since a few years now, two analysis with a three sessions frequency are accepted.*

*To become an ordinary member, you need to*

- *Present an analysis conducted without supervision,*
- *Write a theoretical paper about the case and then present it in front of a commission.*

—

DOI: 10.4324/9781003465409-5

Dear Institute,

My journey as a candidate has been a long and very intense one. Fourteen years of my life, a wedding, a move, two children and the opening of my own practice were all part of it.

I was touched by psychoanalysis when I was eighteen, trying to choose something to study.

The analyst who presented the psychology studies left a deep impression, which was confirmed later while I was sitting in his class. His charisma, the fantasy he made me develop of him being so at ease with himself, so in peace with his drives, convinced me to subscribe. The class he taught was the hilight of my studies.

So, once I was done, I contacted the psychoanalytical Institute I found in my region, full of questions and wondering what the conditions would be. The only thing that came back was a thick envelope. What I understood of the requirements was overwhelming. I felt totally alone and didn't think for a second that anyone on the other side of that envelope might be interested in me. I was not yet 25, doing a few years of internships that were barely paid, working half-time to pay the rent of my little studio, still depending on my parents for my insurances. So the requirements of several hundred sessions of analysis, supervision and classes seemed so totally out of reach that I turned away, and spent the next few years trying out other approaches.

Had anyone actually talked to me, reassured me about the expectations and the timeline to get there, it would maybe have been different. But even now, I have the impression that there is a "too young" to become a candidate, which I think is a problem. They might be too young to become a member, but training takes time anyway, especially in Switzerland.

Now that I have come so far, I wonder. Couldn't whoever send me this envelope have picked up a phone to talk to me? Advise me on how to proceed?

Gladly for my becoming an analyst, the other therapeutic experiences didn't convince me at the core of myself.

So, after three years, I subscribed for a Master in psychoanalytical psychotherapy, in Zurich, which was not only at the other end of our small country, but also the German speaking part of it. My luck was to have been born there and be fluent in Swiss German. It was the only official Master in psychoanalytical therapy taught at a university at that time. For a year, I traveled every two week-ends, sleeping in some stranger's bed because money was tight and my brother had a friend who did the opposite journey, going back to Lausanne on Friday evening. I finally got my first real and ok payed job as a psychologist closer to Zurich, and two years later, I started working as a psychotherapist in training in Zurich.

Having spent my first salary on furniture for my first real apartment – it actually had a bedroom and a living room – I started putting money aside every month for analysis. Many of the teachers of my Master were analysts, and so I had allowed myself to believe it was possible to actually get there.

Soon after having signed my contract for the job in Zurich, a few months before moving there, I went to meet my future analyst. I had been to other first meetings before her, but it never had felt quite right. That was at the time quite difficult, to actually say "no" to a training analyst, even though it was clear for me after the first encounter. My idealization of the "Jedi" as I called them in secret, was strong. I wasn't at ease at all. Knowing they were part of the people who would one day judge my ability to become an analyst didn't make it any easier. During my whole time as a candidate, only one of my supervisors actually clearly stated that our first meeting was for me to see if I wanted to go on working with him.

The next step was to become a candidate. I met with two analysts. The first of them was very easy and agreeable, I came out lighthearted and felt encouraged to continue. But the second interview left me deeply troubled. He wanted more from me than just making sure I wasn't psychotic. He didn't let me off the hook until I accepted to talk about myself, really. But I was also very impressed with his analytical skills, which I discovered applied on myself. He wanted insight, not just enthusiastic talk about my learnings. So after a year, I went back to see him for the second interview. It felt like the challenge I had to take up.

I started classes in the following autumn, and supervision with him two years later, which became a very important part of my training. His clinical skills and his calm way of helping me grasp what was happening in my sessions opened many doors for me.

Half a year later, I went to my first IPSO event. I was deeply touched by the spirit of this event, the long and lively conversations, the ease I saw my colleagues have with each other. The mixture of intellectual stimulation, the pleasure of meeting each other, the trust that grew rapidly. The intimacy of some conversations and the party time was liberating. It was so much easier than what I mostly knew from home.

I consider myself lucky to have gone through the theoretical part of my training in Zurich at a time where there was a special class for candidates. Those of us who joined – many younger ones like me – would all meet every Monday evening for four years, with a few candidates ending and a few new starting every year. But we were a group, we had supervision together, we studied and some of us went for a drink after class. This gave me the feeling of belonging which I hadn't felt when I just picked one or the other seminar at the institute. It was difficult to meet the others, I was too impressed by their knowledge and age, and by the fact that I didn't know who was a fellow candidate and who was already a member. There had been no meet and greet event, no one to help me navigate the crowd. Is it so difficult to welcome the newbies?

I've learned later on that it can be quite a challenge to have candidates meet and build something together. Maybe because many of us are at an age where you can and want to be fully engaged professionally. As you can't do it in psychoanalytical society (members only), you get involved somewhere else. We all have a job and are part of other professional associations, where we have a say, a position.

The very real prize to pay for my training was years of a student-like life-style, at an age at which most of my "normal" friends had a decent salary and no children yet, freedom in many other ways.

I have seen several candidate colleagues give up on training, or struggling really hard, because they had families to care for. My boss in my first years of training was often up to two weeks late with paying the salaries, and when I complained I was told that I should maybe reconsider my choice if I was too anxious to be in a liberal profession. And when I then once couldn't pay for my supervision in time, I was asked if I thought my supervisor deserved to be the one paying for my difficulties.

I chose to train in psychoanalysis, but I have felt very lonely sometimes, and have been very hurt or angry at those who would only serve me an inter-pretation, when I needed a little understanding and some consideration for my reality. Especially from those who have been there.

My husband could sing a song, as goes a saying in German, about the years of that life that he shared with me. First adapting his holiday budget to mine, then paying two-thirds of our first common rent, paying for almost eve-rything once our first child was born and I was not only working a bit less but still paying for four sessions of analysis and two to three hours of supervision per week, spending most of my money on my training. I hated to be in that position, but I am still grateful he never asked me to choose.

What he did, though, was giving me, when needed, the reality kicks to get along with the training, to think and talk about the ending of my analysis and later on to find the courage to present myself in front of the commission.

This is a very difficult moment, at least in the candidate's fantasies. It for sure was in mine. Throughout all of my candidacy years we would hear echoes about colleagues who failed, but as we didn't have access to the information (members only). It was only rumors, sayings, stories. I have envied my IPSO colleagues who would send pictures of themselves on our WhatsApp group, being so confident that after years of training, they were just about to "get in". There was not much doubt about that fact. Whereas we would rarely talk about it, the anxiety being too strong. And for a lot of my companions, finding two patients for analysis was a big difficulty as well, and still is. There is not much done to help candidates find patients. There was a seminar where we would share the phone of the institute and see the people who called, but it seldom brought patients for analysis. From the roughly 15 people of my class, only very few have become members, and I finished ten years ago. It might be the difficulty of a small country, where the local institutes are too small to be able to offer more structured help to find patients for analysis. It was an important recognition of the dif-ficulty of finding patients in present times, to lower the number of sessions per week from four to three for the control cases. Before this decision, I've heard more than once that it was only the candidate's difficulty and needed more personal analysis.

I was a young candidate for Swiss standards, I am now a rather young member, even though I graduated at 45. I have wondered why there was such a difference between my comrades and I and the graduates of the first generations in Europe, who would become members in their early thirties. When Psychoanalysis seemed to be this adventure you could join at a young age and without that many difficulties.

It might be that the difficulty lies within us, that a severe superego has expectations that are too high. But the fact that candidates don't have access to the statistics of the exam, for example, nourishes the fantasies. It also is a fact that it is by far the longest and most expensive training, with for us here in Switzerland this uncertainty that you will actually succeed at the end. When I talk about this with my friends who work in other fields, they shake their head in disbelief.

Last but not least, having to convince thirteen people in less than an hour of one's aptitude is a scary challenge. Eight, ten, often more years of training evaluated in such a manner is frightening. Will the thumb go up or down? Am I really, REALLY ready for that?

Since I got pregnant the first time, it has been a balance that is not always easy to find, between family life and psychoanalysis. It started with the pregnancy. What to do or say when a patient (my first on the couch!) doesn't seem to notice the belly which was so visible? I intended to take a six-month leave after giving birth, so it needed time to be analyzed. Both my supervisors advised me to stay silent. I ended up being so worried that I talked about it in my analysis. It was difficult for me to challenge my supervisor's recommendation. I have no doubt today that they would have talked it through with me to help me, but at the time I was too submissive to be able to clearly voice out my discomfort without the comfort of my analyst in my back. It was after all my first control case, what did I know . . . ?

What to do when a child is sick and can't go to daycare? Stay at home or not? When the teachers need parents to go ice skating with the whole class? Those moments have been quite lonely, when I was confronted with my motherhood intruding my practice. I had ended my analysis during the second pregnancy and moved back to Lausanne. There came this superego conflict, I thought I should be as reliable as possible as an analyst, and I have often chosen to go to work. My own mother taking over most of the time in those situations made it easier on me, but after all, I was in pole position to know what damage an absent mother can do. And would I really be present for my patients?

Once during an IPSO meeting with two experienced and famous analysts, one of them voiced clearly her thought about third-party childcare having a negative effect on the children's growth. I couldn't believe what I had heard and asked again to be sure. There I was, carrying my working mum's guilt, listening to this woman telling us we should attend to our children instead of giving them into the care of others. My worst nightmare, spoken out loud by a teacher of mine – who had no children of her own, one might angrily ad. That is an easy way out of the problem, of course. I realize writing this text that I would have benefitted from a safe place where those concerns could be discussed. Ours is a peculiar journey, and a peculiar job. Maybe we should think about giving it a peculiar attention as well. Our field is the unconscious, but we have a very real life as well, and it seems to me that we are sometimes quick to only take care of the unconscious or even worse, interpret defensively, or aggressively, in situations where, of course, there are unconscious fantasies, but reality also exists.

My journey was, therefore, also one of des-idealization. A liberating one, in the end. It is relaxing to be less impressed by my elder or more experienced colleagues. I had to give up my secret fantasy of becoming like Yoda one day but accepting that there was no Jedi actually makes it easier also on myself. It hasn't changed my sadness to see experienced and sometimes famous colleagues treat each other with such disrespect that it is painful to actually be in the same room.

But I feel confident now that I can participate in the life of my own psychoanalytical society.

As to the two institutes that trained me, I learned that the people actually constituting them are fellow humans, and the more I de-idealized the profession and met actual people, the more I have come to feel part of them. I will always treasure my Ipso memories, and I know I've made friends for life there, but I can also enjoy to talk and dance with my colleagues here in tiny Switzerland.

— Brigitte Dodge

# 6  A letter to the Indian Psychoanalytical Society, Kolkata (1922)

*Gagandeep Kaur Makkar*

*The Indian Psychoanalytical Society was founded in Calcutta (by Girindra Sekhar Bose, in his home) in 1922, just three years after the British Psychoanalytical Society was formed. It was. The Indian Psychoanalytical Society is affiliated with the International Psychoanalytical Association. Mr. Bhupendra Desai (who studied with Bose) and Mr. Amrith contributed largely to the development of psychoanalysis and psychoanalytical training in Bombay (Mumbai). Mrs. Ferny Mehta, another pioneer, headed the Indian Council of Mental Hygiene, an organization that employed Psychiatric Social Workers to lecture and counsel in numerous schools and colleges in Mumbai. In 1974, a group of psychoanalysts founded a public charity trust called the Psychoanalytic Therapy and Research Centre.*
  *For qualifying:*

- *We are expected to present two papers, one based on the clinical work we have done under the supervision and the other on the theoretical topic.*
- *Also, we are expected to see two adult cases minimum under the supervision and the cases must be analytically seen three to four times a week for a reasonable period where unconscious is significantly explored.*

—

14, Parsi Bagan Lane is the lane by the side of the University of Calcutta, where I did my training in Clinical Psychology. The street somehow was always an attraction for me. Standing at the beginning of this lane, I always felt deep. I now can say that it was symbolically an invitation to get inside the hidden shelves of my mind. I was unaware that this particular lane had a historical address—where Psychoanalysis first started in India and Asia.

One fine day, after my university lecture, I took a plunge to fathom the appeal of this lane. The lane where my beloved Institute is magnificently standing did not disappoint me. To get there, I walked past the old traditional houses with trees inside the courtyard of those houses on my right while the massive wall of Calcutta University with branches of the campus trees fell onto

DOI: 10.4324/9781003465409-6

the lane on my left. It was surreal for me. The silence of the lane was therapeutic. This lane and the area around it have significance for being a place for the Parsi community and a reference to the pre-independence era. The Calcutta University premises, and its building are also some 160 years old. After walking some 50 meters, I stood outside the house whose address and name were written on an ancient nameplate. It read Indian Psychoanalytical Society (IPS) 14, Parsi Bagan Lane; now a 100-year-old building constructed in a tropical colonial style. I saw a man coming outside of this building. I was curious and hence stopped that person and asked, what is this place? 'He replied it's a place for looking at the mind.' Looking at the mind, that sounded so interesting. I went back, and the next day, I asked one of my beloved teachers, Late Mr. Arup Ghosal, a psychoanalyst himself, about IPS. He quickly picked up my curiosity and convincingly told me that this is where you will find answers for yourself—Self. I felt that his statement was inviting. With his encouragement and my unconscious curiosity about Parsi Bagan lane, I enrolled as an affiliate of IPS to unravel the secret chambers of my mind. The inside premises of IPS, especially the library, had a magical appeal. The smell of old books, journals, and magazines was addictive. IPS was like Hogwarts for me and became my love. My romance with IPS was in full bloom. Almost every day after my university classes, I would attend classes, psychiatry clinics, supervision, and read in the library. I believe it was only me, but my peers also long for the tea made by Sufol Da, samosas (a savory), and sandesh (a traditional Bengali Sweet) served in Saturday classes. This place gave me the nurturance equivalent to the warmth and love of a mother. I have always felt the premises of IPS to be homely. The analyst and psychiatrist visiting the Institute were warm, welcoming, and, most importantly, nurturing. In formal and non-formal ways, they all taught us the intricacies of the human mind and behavior. My feelings for IPS have evolved from infantile love to a relationship of equality. I feel responsible for giving back to my Institute the love, care, and stability it helped me to achieve for myself. Without IPS, I would not have even gotten this opportunity to write.

Dear Indian Psychoanalytical Society (IPS),

I am opening up to you to describe what I feel about you, my training, and where I emotionally stand today. In doing so, I am speaking my mind out with this faith that you had instilled in me about you that I have been/and will be heard talking about my journey. When I began training in Psychoanalysis, I was not articulate about my expectations from this journey. I went ahead with full conviction for two reasons. Firstly, I will find answers about myself, as Arup Sir told me. Second, I was in awe of my future analyst—Ms. Sarala Kapoor.

My informal conversations at Institute convinced me she was the right one for me. While reflecting, I feel I was choosing the right mother for myself—a warm and available mother. Arup Sir suggested I get my analysis done under

Dr. Pushpa Mishra, who later became my supervisor—and was ideally suited for this role in my training. It took me real guts to tell my beloved teacher that I would like to go ahead with Ms. Kapoor and not Dr. Mishra.

Dr. Mishra is the top pick by the candidates; she is a fulbright scholar and a renowned academician and clinician in the city of Kolkata. I am so glad that Arup sir did not burden me with what he thought was best for me. He respectfully allowed me the free space to exercise my choice.

My training with my analyst was deep. I had moments of awe, falling apart, and hatred toward my analyst. It started with blind love and dependency on her. My analyst gave me a haven to talk and explore. It allowed me to be the child and grow mentally into an adolescent and now as an adult. The journey was not easy, however. We also had our sessions having enactment that made me think if I was the only one having positive and negative transference.

I started to experience jealousy when my peers from the university also began their analysis with my analyst. My analyst told me that I was having a sibling rivalry, which appeared to be a plausible explanation, considering I am the first child of my parents. It was my first encounter with difficult emotions. I soon began to understand how I have denied my experiences and feelings all my life. I was living my life robotically, not knowing the emotional world inside me. I remember telling my analyst how I desired to be part of the olden times when everything was black & white. She replied that the world always had colors and that it was my perception of the world as black & white and not otherwise. There were many moments of deep reflection and insight. Both my analyst and I were happy with each other. I was pleased, as I felt contained. My analyst was delighted, as I was the perfect patient exploring the unconscious seven times a week and coming for sessions from far away on time.

The scenario changed mainly for me when my analyst felt that I had transference resistance, which I felt was my analyst's inability to contain and help me explore my extremely vulnerable side. This was the most challenging phase for both of us. Quite a few sessions went in either silence or intense arguments. I am not sure if this should have happened at all. Perhaps not—at least the arguments. I felt my analyst was distant and inhumane in pointing me my vulnerabilities. It was only later that we took a break to reflect and assimilate what was going on; I could see that my paranoid guards were on an all-time high. Hence, it made me highly critical of her methods and interventions.

Before I made peace with my inner toil, I suffered during this phase. The emotional toll was visible on my physical health too. I lost a lot of weight and ran a low-grade fever for a year. No one understood what was wrong. I was suffering silently and desperately looking for answers because I genuinely felt violated by my analyst. A part of it now I know was my internal structure, and another part was the contribution of my analyst. Her technique to handle paranoid emotions evolved with me. We later got a chance to sort this out, and I am so obliged that she admitted where she went wrong.

Before this happened, as I mentioned, I was struggling and looking for answers. Around this time, International Psychoanalytical Studies Organization—my dear IPSO arrived in my life. I had no idea what it was and how it functions, but it played a significant role in helping me navigate my emotional struggle. I remember attending the first business meeting of IPSO at the 48th International Psychoanalytical Association (IPA) Conference in Prague in 2013. Everyone was so warm and welcoming. Most importantly, I felt they were non-judgmental—critical judgment was what I was struggling with internally. I got the chance to learn about being an IPSO rep, and honestly, I secretly admired being one then. I did not have the courage and faith in myself. I distinctly remember the dynamicity of that room. I felt different there. I will not say happy, but it was different from my usual feeling of somberness.

With this different feeling, I muster the courage to speak to Dr. Samuel Zysman, my supervisor, for the IPSO Clinical Supervision event. I was already in touch with him regarding the supervision. I approached him to have a personal meeting with him. He was kind enough to give me ample time to listen to my concern patiently during the conference. He was empathetic, helped me understand my difficulty, and arrived at a perspective to work on. What I cannot forget about our meeting and my fundamental learning to date is his respect for boundaries and room for the other's perspective. He told me, Gagandeep, take this assertively with your analyst, as you both know the best of what is happening between the two of you in analysis. She may not be the best, but if she listens to you, you know she is genuine; this sometimes is enough.

This answered many unsettled questions, demands, and apprehensions about my analysis, life, and, of course, my analyst. On my return, I continued my relationship with IPSO, as I gradually felt better and better. I could find my voice with peers across the globe. I felt alive again and felt that I was out of my cage. I also went to my analyst and discussed my concerns. We disagreed, but she listened to my concerns and remained firm that I must reflect more. I also told her about my interaction with Dr. Zysman. She interpreted my overstepping the boundaries but understood why I needed to do so. It helped, and I could feel she was genuine. The analysis went ahead, and we could work together and arrive at a mutual termination point roughly four years later. We stand in a respectful relationship between the overlapping roles of collogues/analyst-analysand. Emotionally, I am at my best. I feel in control and, most importantly, self-aware. When I started, I used to feel vulnerable, dependent and lacking understanding about myself. Psychoanalysis qualitatively changed me as a person. The process helped me bloom and find the best version of myself, although I am still evolving.

What significantly helped me during my training was not only my analysis but also the space I enjoyed with my cohorts both at Indian Society and at IPSO. I remember being together with my inner group—Bharti Jain and Jheelum Poddar; having endless discussions on varied topics ranging from books, politics, cinema, psychopathology, and psychoanalytic treatment. We sometimes also discussed the theoretical orientation and the technique used by our analysts and supervisors. The lens of discussion of any topic remained psychodynamic in nature. Our frank and long discussions shaped my analytical thinking—psychoanalytic and analytical.

The teachings of Dr. Salman Akhtar also shaped my training. Dr. Akhtar visited our Institute and gave a lecture on analytic settings. His lecture was like storytelling. His clarity on pathology and ways to penetrate the layers of the mind was quite insightful. I started following his lectures on YouTube, reading his articles, and correspondence with him on areas of difficulty. He was generous enough to help me with my long queries. His working and thinking style shaped the way today I think and practice.

Somewhere during the middle of my analysis, I started my supervision with my supervisor Dr. Pushpa Mishra. She was very different from my analyst and my personality. The first time I saw her, I was apprehensive of her judgment. Fear of judgment was one of my core problems. I thought she would be very strict and rude. To my surprise, I found her to be an elegant older woman with poise and a charming smile that was barely visible. Unlike my analyst and Arup Sir, I was watchful of my behavior with her. I wanted to impress her, but I failed quite a time only for my better. Her therapeutic technique, orientation, and analytical frame were quite different from my analyst's and mine. It took me quite some time to figure out the right balance in my technique by being mindful of my strengths and limitations. A few of her observations about me, such as that I talk too much during my sessions and that it interferes with the analytical space of my client, were challenging to work with. I had to work hard to understand my unconscious need to do so.

Supervision with Dr. Mishra helped me clip the extras of my life and extras in analysis with my patients. In a true sense, I began to understand the value of the minimum, optimum, just, and objective. Her calm demeanor helped me calm my restlessness and extra energy, which was unnoticed by me. I found her to be honest and genuine in helping me be a better analyst. Toward the end of our work together, she encouraged me to write as she felt I was original in my clinical understanding and technique. Unfortunately, despite her guidance and assurance to help me, I still could not do much about my writing skills. I hope that someday, I will be able to impress her with my writing quality—does it sound infantile? Maybe, but I do feel that way.

As a supervisor and seminar instructor, she gave much importance to writing about our understanding of the topic we were taught. Since I was not good at writing and could not improve it, I felt ashamed. The capacity to write was fundamental for my supervisor, is what I thought. I was failing her. Unfortunately, she could never see this. I am sure she would have supported me in working on my inability if I had made an effort. The feeling of shame got aggravated when another, or to be specific, one of the peers, was given several chances to write and present the work at different forums. At that time, it felt discriminatory, but that particular peer was good and got the opportunity.

It was difficult for me to make peace with what appeared to be biased. I was envious of that peer for taking the privileges offered. I never opened up about this to my supervisor. I knew that my peer deserved the chance to be good at writing and clinical work. I could be, too, but I was not. Still, I am not. Accepting reality is quite painful, as I understood. Once accepted, it changes things for the better. My analyst helped me endure this pain to some extent.

I must mention that, once again, what helped me surpass my fear of being bad at writing was the support of one of my dear IPSO collogues, Monica Bomba. Monica offered me the chance to be the discussant for the opening paper of the European Psychoanalytic Federation (EPF) in 2021. I told her I would love to be on board, but I was apprehensive as I am not good at writing. What she said stayed with me. She told me I must not worry about my writing. We all are learning and growing together, and it was mainly about what I feel. Such a beautiful thought conveyed with warmth helped me get the courage to pen down my feelings. I was once again starting to write. Had IPSO not been in my life during my training, I would have been very different, and indeed not for the best. One of the admirable aspects of IPS was that it helped me connect with IPSO. IPS may not have provided the best training at its premise, but it never hindered my growth anywhere possible.

As a batch, we were lucky to have theoretical classes with some senior analysts. We all experienced a change in our understanding of the subject. I could connect to the International vocabulary used by my peers and renowned analysts worldwide. Although, I wish and now strongly feel that the theoretical lessons could have started earlier in training. I still think about this gap in myself. I also contributed to this situation, as I needed to read more, which I was not doing. The training module—both theoretical and clinical at IPS needs to be structured. We are a 100-year-old society thriving on our rich heritage and the goodness of senior analysts. Sadly, that is not enough for society to run for another 100 years.

It irks me to see some of the candidate's casual and capitalistic approach toward psychanalysis in Indian Society. Despite all criticism and challenges, Psychoanalysis has survived due to its strong foundation in the discovery of the unconscious and by the conviction and passion of the people practicing it. Hence, it is not justified to take it as an option for the additional qualification because it is attractive and available besides Calcutta University or can create inroads for practicing therapy. I believe a system has to be in place at IPS, inviting young people to take this profession, but with love, care, and integrity.

The current scenario at IPS is struggling to find pointers on which it can anchor its existence for another 100 years. We need to find answers on why we could not have theoretical training running on auto mode. True, we do not have enough teachers and able administrators. Why is it so that those we have are not able or interested? Why do we not have enough representation in International journals? Is it only the number of qualified analysts from India? I may be wrong, but I feel that we lack a sense of belongingness and gratitude towards the society that gives psychological existence to all thriving analysts. I wonder, where do we stand in our emotional world without gratitude? I know my writing skills are not excellent, but as Monica says, it is about what one feels. Why, as a collective, can we not encourage voices? I do not think my society is not encouraging, but perhaps we are not together in true spirit.

No doubt, the current administration has achieved a few milestones. They have made a 100-year-old library digital. We all rejoiced when the society organized monthly seminars which invited renowned analysts from all over the world for its candidates and members to commemorate 100 years of IPS. However, what is the vision for another 100 years? The recent initiation of clinical dialogue among all three chapters of society is a significant step toward getting some sense of uniformity and transparency in our clinical practice; otherwise, what happens behind the closed doors of consulting rooms remains unexplored other than privately discussed with respective supervisors. Working together with all three chapters to organize the IPA Asia Pacific Conference in New Delhi is an instrumental step to revive and strengthen the psychoanalytic ethos in our society. The effort to revive our journal Samiksha—*to encourage voices* and make it peer-reviewed is a welcome change. Finally, yet importantly, Indian candidates are now joining IPSO, and members are becoming part of the various IPA International committees, a move needed to get exposure and assimilation into the IPA family.

IPS is indeed working in the right direction, but my humble appeal to its members and candidates is to come forward as a collective to work together to let IPS retain its glorious past. Every effort counts—we cannot leave it only to the executive committee to do work. We need to have a functional system firmly rooted in the ethos of genuineness, openness, and integrity. It was '*this*' spirit that made me fall in love with IPS and psychoanalysis and encouraged me to date to speak my mind. Let us ensure that it continues to appeal to many aspiring analysts walking towards the iconic 14, Parsi Bagan Lane. After all, we not only have the responsibility to take care of IPS but also to save and strengthen the existence of our dear psychoanalysis.

Warmly,

— Gagandeep Kaur Makkar

# 7   Another letter to the Indian Psychoanalytical Society, Kolkata (1922)

*Ashis Roy*

*Editor's note: For a brief history of the Indian Psychoanalytic Institute, and requirements for graduation, please refer to Gagandeep Kaur Makkar's letter.*

—

I was introduced to psychoanalysis at home. I grew up surrounded by books written by Jung and Freud. Born to parents who were psychologists, I would absorb the use of words like the 'shadow' or the 'unconscious'. Freud and his ideas were respected but constantly contentious in an academic setting at the University of Delhi that had cognitive psychologists, industrial psychologists and others who would debate and refute each other's ideas. Within the culture of chaos creativity and passion would pull the student in me in different directions. A wound had been licked and opened and it gave birth to the desire for a deeper absorption within the field of psychoanalysis. Fortunately, the Centre for Psychoanalytic Studies was founded, and I could be a student all over again for the next three years of my life . . .

By this time, I had enrolled into a doctoral program which focused on studying the construction of the Other in inter-faith Hindu-Muslim couples. This lineage translated into the creation of a 'psychosocial-clinical' perspective in Ambedkar University Delhi, where I got involved in the creation and teaching of psychoanalytically informed programs across different academic levels. Later, I invited Sarah Nettleton to speak on the work of Christopher Bollas and this culminated in attending seminars by him at Dartington Hall. Most recently, I was able to organise seminars on the work of Andre Green with Fernando Urribari, who has written on Green and worked with him over years. The Delhi Chapter affiliated to the Indian Psychoanalytic Society organised monthly clinical supervisions where, through the writings of Barranger & Barranger, Ferro, Bion, Tustin, Bergstein, Steiner, clinical processes and the understanding of the 'field' in psychoanalysis became more prominent. They organised a three day seminar with Avner Bergstein which was an unforgettable emotional experience.

DOI: 10.4324/9781003465409-7

Dear Institute,

Looking back to my training I find that the diversity in reading was most helpful in absorbing psychoanalysis as I formally entered training analysis, supervision and simultaneously worked on my doctoral dissertation. My introduction to a range of psychoanalytic writers helped me in reading different 'kinds' of psychoanalysis. In different phases of my life, I found myself to be involved in a deeper learning of different analysts. I spent two years on an online workshop dedicated to the works of Michael Eigen in which people from across the world would read, write and discuss parts of his books. In my supervision with him I learnt how a deeply intuitive supervisor can stimulate the unconscious into an aliveness and result in a night full of creative dreaming.

My ongoing training in psychoanalysis made me feel comfortable in different contexts. As I taught courses on psychoanalytic psychotherapy, psychoanalytic research and on working with states of disintegration I re-absorbed what I had studied in my formative years and developed a deeper relationship. It became easier to create within the students an ongoing relationship with different kinds of psychoanalytic writing – a relationship that had been created for me by my teachers. Similarly presenting in national and international conferences gave me more confidence to write and feel comfortable with my ideas. As I met other candidates, I learnt that studying in the university gave me a wider breadth in understanding psychoanalysis and not prematurely aligning myself with schools of psychoanalysis. As I trained with the Indian Psychoanalytic Society they appreciated and were open to this diversity. Each member was affected in deeply emotional ways as unformulated experiences penetrated everyone, which was remarkable.

I was fortunate to be in a system which had an interface between an interdisciplinary university setting and different Psychoanalytic societies across the world. In part I created this system as I organised and participated in several cross cultural international psychoanalytic conferences with Germany, France and Japan. Each conference had a cultural and clinical focus, and the best writer was awarded the Sudhir Kakar award. I was fortunate to win the Critics award in the Indo-Japan conference which was presented to me by the esteemed analyst Mr. Kitayama.

Along with working with patients three/four times a week, I was fortunate to develop a sensitivity to low fee clinical work for marginalised communities that could not afford therapy at the university clinic in Ambedkar University. A social sciences university enabled me to think of subjecthood and marginality in a variety of ways. I could closely engage with students in the classroom as courses in psychoanalysis opened their internal worlds and simultaneously, I could engage with the conflicts and internal worlds of other students in the clinic. I developed a closer understanding of a life stage that transitions from adolescence to adulthood and needs a moratorium before it gains a distinctive identity. As a teacher, students would often ask— you have unpacked our internal worlds and how do we pack it back? Although in the clinic via holding, containing and interpretation we help the patient, in the classroom it was difficult to provide the same holding environment to the students. For them, psychoanalysis initiated a new journey into selfhood, which was undulating for the student even though it was also enriching and insightful. Subsequently, some students would pursue further training in psychoanalysis, and many would work as counsellors and therapists in schools, colleges and in private practice.

Thus, my exposure to Psychoanalysis benefitted from being situated within a university and being a part of an institute. The university gave me the opportunity to participate in organisational building and development. The experience of being supervised by Michael Eigen and Neil Altman (USA), Pumpi Harel (Israel), Renato Trachenberg (Brazil), Mallika Akbar (India) exposed me to different traditions in psychoanalysis. Simultaneously, my clinical work involved working with varying cultural realities in my country. This interface helped my work in developing a nuanced understanding of Queer, Muslim, Catholic and socio-economically disadvantaged patients.

In retrospect, my training and understanding of psychoanalysis made me deeply curious about ways of knowing the internal worlds of patients that were object less, fragmented, unformed and unintegrated while simultaneously maintaining an awareness that there were socio-cultural and historical traumas that affected their psychic life as well. Many patients in India suffer from the unprocessed inter-generational trauma, which took place during the Partition of India and Pakistan. It is a divide that remains unmourned in the history of the nation.

Later I was fortunate to be appointed to the faculty at CAPA (Chinese Association for Psychoanalytic Therapy) and started teaching and training CAPA students. It was interesting for me to see how I could sense and work deeply with patients who belong to another culture. A one-and-a-half-day Clinical presentation at the Inter specificity group (at the European Psychoanalytic Federation Conference in Madrid) had given me the exposure of being in a setting where Clinical material could be understood by members from varying cultures. This was another new experience of teaching students who belonged to an older life stage and to a different culture.

Dear institute – as you can see, I have expressed how fortunate I have been, over and over again in this journey. The editor of this book pointed out that I seem to be a confident individual who has taken extra-ordinary initiative to reap his fortunes. Here is my curiosity – how can we help candidates who have not taken this route? Talented candidates who have aspirations desires – just like me – but may not have felt comfortable just stepping up and approaching stalwarts and giants in the industry?

— Ashis Roy

# 8 A letter to the Israel Psychoanalytic Institute, Tel-Aviv (1934)

*Naftally Israeli*

*For the Israel Psychoanalytic Institute, the requirements are:*

- *Completing five years of lectures and seminars (one day per week).*
- *Three cases under supervision (two cases should be four-times-a-week, one can be three-times-a-week, all should be for at least two years in length; each case is supervised by a different instructor; and there is a maximum fee the candidate can ask for each session under supervision—about $60 in Israeli money).*
- *The completion of your own training analysis, which should start when you begin the supervised cases and be four-times-a-week for at least 500 hours (a minimum of about two years and a half in analysis).*
- *Writing a paper which presents one of your cases and receiving an approval of this paper by two instructors who have not supervised you during your studies.*

*Candidates who conduct child-analysis have additional requirements, such as:*

- *Another case under supervision.*
- *Two of their controlled cases should be with analysands under 18 years of age (one teenager and one child).*
- *Additional mandatory lectures and seminars.*

*In Israel there are two psychoanalytic institutions, but only one of them is recognized by the IPA. It was founded in 1934 by Max Eitingon, a favorite student of Freud's, who fled in 1933 from the terror of the Nazis and moved from Berlin to Jerusalem. He bought a beautiful house and dedicated it to the study and practice of psychoanalysis, during his life and after his death. A few years ago, on the edge of a few votes, a decision was made to move the institute from Jerusalem to Tel-Aviv, Israel's cultural center. Today the two institutes, the "Jerusalem-ian" institute and the "Tel-Aviv-ian" one (founded some 20 years ago), are both situated in Tel-Aviv.*

---

DOI: 10.4324/9781003465409-8

Dear Institute,

A few years ago, when I was only vaguely dreaming of analytical training, I visited the Freud Museum in London. I remember my excitement at the sight of the couch, and the instant desire I had to cross over, to pass the marked dividing line and lie on it; or maybe just to sit a little while on the chair behind it. A little later, when I thought more seriously about becoming an analyst, I imagined myself learning together with talented and intelligent people, thirsty for knowledge and full of passion and love for truth. Those unique ones who know a lot about the human soul, always want to know more, and are not afraid to discover hidden truths—both about others and about themselves. In these thoughts, a grandiose childhood phantasy was probably also involved—to be someone great, or to take shelter in the shadow of someone who is (or was) much greater than me. If a psychoanalyst—then like Freud, who, like other people in fields I have always been attracted to (like physics or music), had great passion and courage to change the rules and offer something new. Almost every lecture I hear in psychoanalysis begins with an offering to an ancestor, an offering that wishes to sanctify and please her, and perhaps in this way to allow her spirit to leave in order to allow us to live in the present and to be who we are; to allow us to actually resist her spirit and to say something different, something very personal that is ours. In retrospect, I can say that I have also taken this path: both in my psychoanalytic journey, starting some years ago in the Freud Museum, and in this very text.[1] This is what I probably imagined my psychoanalytical institute will be like, and what it will allow me to become.

But analytical training requires discipline, and discipline—and perhaps alongside it also suppression of spontaneity and impulse—is something which I cultivated from a young age. I kept my grandiose phantasies to myself. I read Freud, I even wrote a PhD related to psychoanalysis, but I didn't dare to start analytical training. Like in the Freud Museum, my internal rule was also clear to me: the couch can only be looked at from a distance. I obeyed, restrained my impulse, so—although I can still imagine the feeling—I cannot tell you what the particular couch in the Freud Museum feels like.

Limiting my internal drive was another reason for the fact that external motivation played an important role in facilitating my decision to study psychoanalysis. For many years I have been working in the Hebrew University's Psychological Clinic in Jerusalem. One day the chief psychologist, who worked there for more than 20 years, called me because he wanted to talk to me about something important. I arranged with him for a Sunday morning meeting, which in Israel is the first day of the week—a difficult hour of traffic jams and organizations for a new week. That morning, I got ready and went to work, arrived at the office just on time, and forgot our meeting. After 20 minutes or so he called me up to ask if I was coming. I was horrified—how could I possibly forget? I thought. "It's not too bad", he said. "Actually, what I wanted to say is very brief: go and study psychoanalysis. I think it will suit you well. I have been debating it for too many years, and I am too old. I have missed the train—don't make the mistake I did". For me it was a precise and special gift, given to me directly from a father-substitute in his sixties, who opened the way for me to become a psychoanalyst by telling me: I believe in you, I see in you a sort of continuation of what I have believed in all these years. You will be able to complete what I have not been able to. I started to imagine that in a psychoanalytic institute, I will find people who will see in me what he already saw. As I live in Jerusalem, I thought these people will be some of my teachers and instructors from this city, in which you, my dear institute, has been since 1934.

But at the time of my registration, when I came to my analysis, the face of my analyst said defeat—the institute will move to Tel-Aviv. Is this really the right time to start studying psychoanalysis, I thought to myself? Precisely now, when my studies will require me to devote an extra 4 hours just to reach the new institute in Tel-Aviv? Isn't this actually a sign of decline of psychoanalysis? Isn't it better to learn another, new, technique of treatment?

At the reception held for us, 1st year candidates, by the 5th year "senior" candidates, I had the opportunity to visit the old house. I was impressed by a beautiful building with a spiral staircase heading up a balcony inlaid with colorful mosaics, and a large painting of Freud at the entrance. But all this was like a dream of Vienna at the beginning of the 20th century. Our classes actually take place every week very close to Tel-Aviv's urban center: between a hamburger shop emitting frying smells and a night bar whose music sometimes overshadows our lecturer's words. From the windows you can see delivery persons on scooters speeding up next to one of the city's expensive malls. When I received the list of my year's candidates, my eye fluttered over their addresses: Tel-Aviv, Tel-Aviv, Tel-Aviv, Tel-Aviv . . . Out of 15 candidates, only three from the periphery of Israel: Myself, from Jerusalem, and two candidates from the north of the country. Israel is a powerful country in terms of psychoanalysis: if there is one analysis per 80,000 people worldwide, in Israel there is one per 10,000—eight times more (Kolke, 2022). If we are already moving outside Jerusalem, I asked myself (and I am now asking you—my dear institute), don't we have an ethical responsibility to take care of the underprivileged? Shouldn't it be more appropriate to place our institute in a peripheral city, outside of Tel-Aviv? Aren't moral considerations more important than the comfort of the majority of the institute's members and candidates, including me?

Having said all this, my dear institute, when I entered your doors I almost immediately fell in love: I felt a strong feeling of belonging to a group of smart, talented, and experienced people; and the teachers seemed to me like those who really understand psychoanalysis, can contribute to my understanding and give me directions. Even now I feel that this "falling in love" is a very important element for me in the training. To connect with the sources of my passion, to love what I do, to admire the people I learn from—all these help me a lot in the labour of learning psychoanalysis, which for me is a daily, Sisyphean and very difficult job. About half of my labour-time is dedicated to it, and my mind is desperately attempting for optimization—eating and driving at the same time, writing late at night, using breaks for other tasks. This is not only a concretization of the psychic burden of the training, and the result of it is an overwhelming feeling, like a plate of food that is overloaded again and again until it can no longer carry the food in it. I want to eat less and less, and give up anything that is not essential or necessary and a "must": conferences, lectures, workshops, seminars . . . All these gifts I leave on my doorstep, preventing myself from bringing them home. Like a monkey who doesn't want to hear, to see, or to know, concentrating only on what is needed to survive. I see the prices my children pay for the personal process I am going through, and the hard work of my wife to hold our family together. During these years I often feel that I just don't have the strength. Sometimes I really hate what I have done to myself. For a brief moment I sometimes think: how hard it is to do what I actually came for—to stop and to look inward, to understand what is happening to me, to stop and ask: Where am I? Who do I want to be? What kind of analyst will I be? How difficult it is to stop and to look. If I could guess, I suppose only a few candidates will stop to read this text, because this action requires unbearable self-observation in the midst of a grueling training, the overt statement of which is "Look at yourself!". In doing so, it immediately produces resistance, a counter pull: "Just don't look!".

This is a major criticism I have, my dear institute: the excessive preoccupation with doing does not allow us essential being, from which meaningful doing can develop (Winnicott, 1971a). It also makes it difficult to "look up", to look at our training in a broader, local, context, and to address social and ethical issues that I feel should be at the heart of our doing. Issues such as the Palestinian problem, the general attitude towards minorities in Israel, discrimination on the basis of gender, ethnicity, or race, the issue of refugees, or the terrible war which was forced this year on Ukraine. The day-to-day burden is too heavy a burden and does not allow me to engage in things that are important to those who specialize in psychoanalysis. It reduces us, candidates, to survival whose basis is fear and obedience to authority and rules and does not direct us to look for our passion and to what is personal. In Hebrew, the word "general" is derived from the same linguistic root as the word "rule", and this connection helps me to formulate what psychoanalysis is for me, and what I think my dear institute misses: psychoanalysis for me deals with passion and the personal, that is, with derivations of love and what is always subversive against what is general, what is stated as a rule. Where are all these in our training? I think that in order to achieve them, we need to be treated not only as apprentices—children who are supposed to undergo regression (an important aspect, which I do not underestimate its value)—but also as responsible adults who are looking for their personal identity and decided to take a journey in order to find it. My membership in IPSO, as one of the Israeli representatives, allowed me to understand this more deeply and from a comparative perspective. I wandered about the many activities organized by other candidates around the world—conferences, seminars, parties, meetings, training, writing, and more . . . Why am I not busy with all this, and why am I similar to the dozens of candidates who study with me at the Israeli institute? In my view, this is a striking point of difference between the Israeli candidates and other candidates worldwide, who, in my opinion, feel much "bigger". My criticism is mainly against the rules that keep us "small" in our institute, against the infantilization of the training process in Israel, and a call to change certain rules in it which will allow the candidates to choose what they study, to study together with candidates from other years and even with analysts, to express themselves more freely, and in general to create who they are going to be instead of imitating what is already known and recognized. I think that changing the rules will allow us, candidates, much more freedom, and will also put a major part of the training "on our shoulders". This, in turn, will help us shape our personal path, and free us from the burden of trying to survive and imitate others who are "bigger" than us. This freedom also requires much more free, non-task time, time of "staring" or "wandering" between different psychoanalytic theories (Benjamin, 1940), getting to know people who have chosen to be psychoanalysts, and, of course, learning from instructors and teachers for many years. The freedom of the kind I am talking about also requires a greater freedom of choice for the candidate, so that he can choose for himself what, with whom, and from whom to study psychoanalytic theory, which is no longer monolithic today.

Compared to this ideal, my dear institute, at the current point where I am now, I feel mostly dissoluted: beyond the identifications and sediments of others (my parents, my siblings, my partner, my children, my friends, my analyst, my teachers, my instructors . . .) it is difficult for me to recognize myself, and it is difficult for me to recognize what therapist I am. What was clear to me until the beginning of my analytical training, suddenly loses form. I find myself identifying with a poet I've always loved—Yona Wallach—but suddenly, her words take on a deep meaning for me. The imperative from one of her poems—about being passive and letting the words do things for you—takes on a frightening reality for me. Death, illness, or madness become real possibilities in the psychoanalytic journey. Words from another one of her poems—about not coming back from an interesting journey you are curious about—ring in my head, as a metaphor for my psychoanalytic excursion. And when I'm back again on the train from Tel-Aviv I feel tired, exhausted. I just want to rest, eat and drink. I feel vulnerable, docile, with thin skin, exposed almost immediately to my pain, and able to easily feel the pain of others. All these pains fail to be completely translated into words, and their residue drains into the body, my body. It feels weaker, sicker, since the training began. My knee begins to hurt. When I look in the mirror, I notice my hair is whitening and waning. Scary thoughts haunt me. I miss Tal, a good friend with whom I played in the past, and after she started analytical training, she got cancer and passed away. Another teacher tells us in class that we need to take care of ourselves, because caring for others can have a negative effect, to the extent that we can actually get sick. When I am flooded by these thoughts, I remember another poem by Yona Wallach, who—like my friend Tal—died from cancer at a young age. This poem talks about the body being smarter than the mind, saying "Enough!" when the mind wants more and more. Could it be that my body is saying something that my mind still doesn't grasp? Does it indicate for me a gap between what my mind wants and what my body can do, a gap that if I miss, I might be in danger?

Another gap I recognize is the gap between myself as an analysand and myself as a future analyst. As an analysand, at the current point in time, I get lost in the tangles of my identifications. I don't know where we are going and what exactly is going to happen. I hold on to my analyst and trust her, feeling small in front of adults who know better than me. A few minutes later, in my clinic and next to my first analysand who feels broken, sick, and desperate, I find myself in a totally different position. He turns to me and asks: "What will the future bring?", and I find myself saying confidently, without knowing where my source of confidence comes from: "I'm with you, whatever will be". He accepts this and then returns again and again to this statement as a beacon that directs the way for him. This gap inside feels, for me, huge, unbearable, sometimes really crazy.

Somehow amongst all these things, islands of my desire and subversion slowly emerge. After many years of Winnicottian instruction, I decided to turn to a Kleinian instructor. The beginning was terrible: a difficult feeling of fragmentation, a disconnection between different training methods, and an impossible feeling in the face of completely opposing instructions, such as "the main thing is that you should be with your patient, experience this moment with him"—as opposed to "the main thing is that you express the separation between you and the patient, and do not give in to the pressure he exerted on you to be with him". Again—a slight feeling of madness. In this "madness" I learned to recognize the subversive moments of my instructors and to learn from them. One of them told me that she was at a conference and was supposed to participate in several workshops, each with a different theoretical approach. But she preferred a certain instructor, and "slipped" into her workshop again and again even though it was actually forbidden. That's how she fell in love with Klein and continued to study and teach her theory all her life. Falling in love and subversion have become for me signs of the subjective, and my ear is attentive to them. "How can one build a subversive theory, a theory that teaches you to break the rules it lays down for you?", I ask myself, and wish you, my dear institute, to tell me how.

A warm place in my heart is reserved for what I understand is unique in Israel—the peer group I study with. We are 15 candidates who started studying together in 2019. The personal, social, and professional meetings with these friends are a great source of pleasure for me. I want to thank each and every one of them—they teach me a lot and allow me to continue on this path that I have chosen to take. The ability to hear other opinions, to know people who are in the same area of development and also a bit whimsy as me, to grumble and gossip with them, to vent aggression, and above all—to simply express myself more freely, without parental "super ego"—all of this benefits me greatly. One of the conversations I remember most from the first year is the conversation about the couch—which couch to buy? Which color? And of course—where? . . . I only vaguely remembered the couch from the Freud Museum, and I chose a couch that reminded me of its color.

One of my guides once told me: she was walking along a narrow path between several houses when suddenly several puppies jumped at her from one of the yards. She was frightened and did not understand why they didn't continue right up to her. She imagined how they would bite her cruelly. But when she looked up, she realized something different happened: their mother, who had also barked at her aggressively, was tied with a rope. She stretched the rope to the limit of her ability, and her puppies stopped there, next to her. The cubs could have continued but they didn't; they understood what their mother's gaze meant, and stopped in an imaginary line, parallel to the rope and near their mother. In this long search for who we are, I understand that we are, first of all, who we are shaped by the gaze of those who observe us—the way we see ourselves in the mirror (Lacan, 1949) and the way we see ourselves in the eyes of our parents (Winnicott, 1971b). Our real and metaphorical parents shape the way for us but limit us in their view. Their anxiety, their pain, their history, which is not exactly ours—all these are limiting. Sometimes our gaze is too focused, for example, when we are too busy with doing, too much focused on a goal, or busy all the time with the way we are perceived by others, or with our parent's anxiety. Sometimes our gaze is too scattered, for example, when we are only busy with observation and associative thought, or when we are disconnected and isolated. One can see the overly focused gaze as arising from high anxiety, and the scattered gaze as one associated with low anxiety. I wish you, my dear institute, would allow us something beyond that, beyond gaze and anxiety: an experience of our self that happens precisely when we manage to get out of these gazes, and experience ourselves in their absence. I know the psychoanalysts in my institute want to share with me and the other candidates the meaningful experience they have, to teach us the psychoanalysis they know, and they do so with great enthusiasm and wisdom. But in order to find our personal selves as analysts, I feel that we also need the opportunity (and the time that will enable it) to deny this view, that is, to deny what we are taught, to rebel against it, and to simply say "No!". Such a possibility would perhaps be the real moment when I would begin to learn a new psychoanalytic thought, a thought that would be mine. I long for this moment.

— Naftally Israeli

## Note

1  Yael Guttel and Inbal Allon-Schindel, together with me, represent the Israeli candidates in IPSO. I wish to thank them for their insightful thoughts and close friendship during the last two years, which helped me formulate the ideas I have expressed here.

# 9 A letter to the Swedish Psychoanalytical Society, Stockholm (1934)

*Eva Christina Tillberg*

*The Swedish Psychoanalytical Society (SPAF) was founded in 1934. The current Swedish Psychoanalytical Association (www.psykoanalys.se)* was formed in 2010 by the joining of SPAF and The Swedish Psychoanalytical Association (SPAS) founded in 1968. Today it consists of 175 psychoanalysts and 30 candidates (23 candidates and 7 post-seminarists, 2022-08-10).

The training at the Swedish Psychoanalytical Institute follows the requirements of IPA according to the Eitingon model. Today, an integrated child-adult training is offered. Eligible to apply is anyone who, at the start of the training, has obtained a degree in psychotherapy, medicine, psychology, or another equivalent academic degree that the Institute assesses in the individual case to fulfill the requirements. Candidates admitted with a medical or psychology degree must have received their license at the end of the training. All candidates must have at least 300 hours work experience in psychiatric practice and at least 150 hours with children and adolescents by the end of the psychoanalytic training. The hours can be assigned to work periods of different length and intensity. Half of these hours must be completed before the candidate begins their first supervised control case. Admission to the education is organized and carried out by the Institute's Admissions Committee. Those who are judged to be eligible are asked to submit a curriculum vitae and will be interviewed by two different interviewers on two consecutive occasions with the respective interviewers. After completed interviews the Admissions Committee proposes admission to the Institute, who makes a decision on admission. For all applicants, experience of own psychoanalysis is desirable at the time of application.

The training at the Swedish Psychoanalytical Institute consists of seminars during 4, 5 years on a weekly basis, clinical psychoanalytic work with three supervised control cases, and a final scientific report/essay on a psychoanalytical subject. The candidate must undergo psychoanalysis with a training analyst with a frequency of 4–5 sessions/week during a minimum of three years. All candidates are recommended to take psychoanalysis during the course of their training. If the candidate has not taken psychoanalysis, it must be started with a training analyst at the latest at the start of the seminars. If the candidate has taken psychoanalysis, it must not have been completed more than five years before the time of admission in order to

DOI: 10.4324/9781003465409-9

be credited. If the candidate has undergone psychoanalysis but not with a training analyst, psychoanalysis must begin with a training analyst at the latest at the start of their supervised control cases. Of the three psychoanalytic control cases the candidate is required to conduct, the first two should run with a frequency of 4–5 times per week and the third with a frequency of 3–4 times per week. For approval, one case must last for three years, one for two years and one for one year. The last can be a psychoanalysis with a child or an adolescent. The individual supervision takes place with a frequency of once per week during the first year and can, in consultation with the supervisor, take place every two weeks thereafter. The Supervisory Committee organizes regular evaluations with the supervisor, candidate and a representative from the Supervisory Committee. The candidate's choice of supervisor must be approved by the Supervisory Committee before the supervision begins. The first case can begin after the first year's seminar teaching has been approved. The candidate agrees not to conduct psychoanalysis beyond the supervised psychoanalyses under the supervision of the Supervisory Committee. Candidates are requested to apply for membership in the Swedish Psychoanalytic Association within six months of completing their training.

—

Dear Institute,

It was a privilege to be accepted to training and undergo this special and profound learning period which has been so rich in content. The aim of the training is to become a psychoanalyst, but I like to think about training as an invitation to search for knowledge and further growth. Psychoanalysis and the training to become a psychoanalyst contain so much more than the learning itself, essentials such as life, friendship and time. As an Institute for training you gave me the opportunity to (re-) connect to and further learn from the psychoanalytical legacy. You provide this particular learning space for me. It is essential in your role as an Institute, I think, to take care of the psychoanalytical legacy and pass it on.

Dear Institute, I address you from the other side of the seminar period in my new candidate role as a post-seminarist. I no longer belong to a weekly based seminar group. Training proceeds for some time still though, with the supervised clinical cases. Shortly after the seminar training period had ended, I was invited to contribute to this collection of letters. Our final theses had recently been written, presented and discussed in the group of experienced psychoanalysts within The Swedish Psychoanalytical Association. It was a special event that made me feel welcomed into a larger scientific and social context. The invitation to write a letter addressed to my Institute connected to this phase of training and brought the possibility to reflect upon what training means so far and what you as an Institute represent.

Dear Institute, let me say something about the form of this text. It is defined as a letter, the well-known form of communicating that involves two (or several) subjects in the modality of the written word going from a specific sender to a specific receiver. It indicates something personal. However, this specific letter involves not just the two of us but aims at being read by many others. You might say it is addressed to "everyone and nobody", which in a sense is something quite anonymous. Initially I thought about questions such as if the Institute could be considered a subject and how could a glimpse of my personal point of view of training be of interest to a wider audience? I am a candidate at this Institute, but I also belong to the global network of candidates. During training I have gained experience and knowledge from outside your direct Institute sphere. The contact with candidates from other Institutes around the world has brought a multifaceted perspective to training. This has broadened my view of classical and contemporary psychoanalysis and how different training cultures and traditions shape us. The answer to my initial question about what possibly could be of a general interest to the reader would be: that it is the collection of letters to our respective Institutes that form a pluralistic image of what it means to be a candidate in progress today. This extended context symbolizes personal growth and the privilege to develop.

Dear Institute, in this new phase of training, my fellow candidates and I have become the older sibling leaving home, reshaping ourselves in a process of reduced dependence and increased independence. Training groups following ours are your current focus for attention. To reach this phase in training has required a profound work from my side, and from yours. I mentally digest the total situation as training proceeds in a changed form, speed and rhythm. Being neither just a candidate in the former sense, nor a full member psychoanalyst, is sensed as a Winnicottian potential space that can promote change. Whether it was your intention or not, it offers new experiences of being a candidate when slowly embodying a new identity.

Dear Institute, occasionally I miss the regular seminar context you provided. We had time and space to read, think, talk, write and learn together in a creative room for the mind at work. This was one important reason why I eventually decided to apply to training—to take care of my mind at work. Psychoanalysis and psychoanalytic thinking were and had been under severe external pressure in Sweden for a longer period. Something essential was at risk of being weakened or even get lost. I guess the Swedish Psychoanalytical Association and you, its Institute, were affected by these anti-psychoanalytical winds blowing through society as well. Nevertheless, you were still there. The almost forgotten vague dream to apply to psychoanalytic training one day in the future came to surface. I imagined a large and crowded family united by a shared interest gathered under a common umbrella. The initial welcome meeting in the Old Town of Stockholm gathered representatives from the Institute, and my fellow candidates that would become our joint training group. The situation was new and still I sensed a feeling of homecoming, something familiar. The Old Town of Stockholm with its buildings and streets founded in the 17th century formed a physical-psychical base for training located on historical ground. I felt at home.

Dear Institute, you apparently represented what a home feels like. What does that mean? Obviously it is not only about the physical external structure consisting of walls, floors, ceiling and furniture, but rather about the physical in connection with psychic aspects in terms of form, memory and narrative. Aspects of emotionality interact with the physical shaping a multifaceted psychic web of meaning. Another personal image that relates to home to me is of a river with its origin springing from an ancient source. It floats through a constantly changing landscape in a clear direction. Whirls, streams, sudden and opposite shifts, eddies and meanders expresses unexpected qualities which can be harsh and difficult to handle, or show soothing kindness or dynamic force. Sidebanks hold the flow containing its circuits. Cities, villages and houses appear and disappear, locations that gather people living their ordinary daily lives. The internal experience corresponds with the external in linking vital elements together, a balance of containment of uncertainty and security. This metaphor connects to the psychoanalytic dream. Embedded in the project of training lies the search for, and the finding of, the internal world—the unconscious. Dreaming the training is thus one way to connect to it.

Dear Institute, by investing in such a huge project as psychoanalytic training I did not only put myself in contact with dreaming but with reality as well. Training involved a number of crises, or revolutions. The Latin *revolutio*, " a turn around", can be understood as a notion of crisis. Before starting the first term we were introduced to the summer reading of "Revolution in mind—the creation of psychoanalysis" (Makari, 2009). You presented us a splendid starting spark that evoked my curiosity. This beautiful and dynamic narrative of uncertainties mixed with a passionate search for knowledge are components that represent good companions and cooperation partners when entering unknown terrains. To start training in this way initiated the importance of the history of ideas, their origin and how they evolve over time; theory as a living materia. Conflictual interests were described, possible to relate to when embarking on the training project. To deal with conflict was a vital ingredient to make training possible and durable. The very beginning of training could thus be understood as a (first) training crisis. A second training crisis appeared after about a year, facing the quite vulnerable position of starting supervised control cases. My professional identity as an experienced and senior psychoanalytical psychotherapist was challenged. I could well relate to the clinical situation as such, but I perceived psychoanalysis as something different; I just couldn't figure out quite in what way. Ambivalence, hesitation and doubt that psychoanalysts in general and candidates in particular feel when beginning this full-scale commitment was well captured by Ehrlich (2012). Her article "The analyst's reluctance to begin a new analysis" highlighted dilemmas, offered recognition, inspiration and hope. The two above mentioned texts addressed me directly as a candidate beginning training. Through your seminar committee your choice of the mentioned literature is an example of how you seemed to encourage me to embark on the training journey itself. As time passed and training became more integrated, a third crisis arose: the COVID-19 pandemic struck nationally and world-wide.

Dear Institute, this crisis was of a different quality. It didn't relate to a maturational crisis within the training situation but had more of a traumatic quality initiated from external pressure. The training structure changed overnight, and we suddenly found ourselves reduced to small squares in a corner of the computer. A flat screen showing my teachers, candidate peers and myself as talking heads constituted a dramatic shift in the psychic learning atmosphere. The first months conducted exclusively digitally on Zoom were quite painful from my point of view. The sudden loss of the on-site reflective containment space for psychoanalytical thinking felt sad. The situation changed the way psychoanalytical knowledge just recently had been perceived and taken in. Hesitations about continuing training grew as I slowly realized I couldn't benefit from learning only via technology modality. Overlooking a longer period it seemed impossible and was far away from the original reason why I had chosen to apply, and accept going into, training. I am well aware of that in some parts of the world technology was the only solution. Over here there was still a small opportunity for alternatives. Eventually you offered seminars in a hybrid form. It took some time for you to reach, but it absolutely saved my training process.

Dear Institute, through your teachers, supervisors, course coordinators, seminar committee, supervision committee and the principal, I know you did what was possible to try to overcome the problems this situation caused. I know you struggled to keep training running uninterrupted, trying hard to make necessary adjustments. But to be a candidate means being in a vulnerable position and being dependent. I lacked your felt presence during this initial time of sudden shift. There wasn't always new information to give of course, but it would have been valuable with some kind of resonance from you, a recognition of the total situation, your personal voice. Maybe a weekly written letter? I can't articulate exactly what. Why would your voice be so important? Maybe because training is demanding in so many ways. Framework and structures are crucial to make it possible. It's not just about the manifest frame but about the internal frame. This particular sound of silence touched upon primitive states of mind such as helplessness and abandonment.

Dear Institute, we all faced the terrible pandemic situation, not being able to connect or to meet our loved ones in person as we were used to. To undergo training during these circumstances was a challenge. The specificity of the psychoanalytical work is in some sense a lonely position. As psychoanalysts and psychotherapists, we give so much of ourselves to our patients and we need nourishment, support and inspiration from a scholarly and social context. Neither you nor me had a map for how to handle this viral attack that touched upon primitive states of mind. I consider this a shared crisis from our different roles and perspectives. Eventually, we psychologically survived with mutual effort.

Dear Institute, I know you drew conclusions from the experiences of this period and I know you protect the value of on-site training. The importance of on-site training is, from my point of view, not interchangeable with learning psychoanalytical knowledge through technology. The Zoom seminars created uneasy feelings linked to learning, which partly might be connected to the length of the seminars. The length of seminars suited the on-site form well but became tiresome on-line. I feel grateful I encountered the physical form for quite a long time before the context changed. Technology is tempting in its easiness to use, like if only a concrete switch from one modality to another would be the solution to a complex problem. The possibility to use technology as an emergency solution is still good enough, and invaluable compared to if there isn't any alternative. I do think psychoanalytical knowledge can be transferred through technology, but I think it might need to adjust to the form and media through which it is presented—it could be a matter of didactics.

Dear Institute, I end my letter with some reflections upon the subtle but indisputable difference between the psychotherapist and psychoanalyst. This theme has leapt like a thread through my training, starting as a psychotherapist who will finish as a psychoanalyst. You highlighted the distinctions and presented theoretical material on the subject, like e.g., through Blass (2010). These lines of thoughts brought forward different perspectives regarding distinctions and technique. With references to Busch, Kächele and Widlöcher, Blass highlighted the importance of dialogue over controversial issues rather than the resolution of them, which I find encouraging and a fresh approach to understand theory and clinical practice. Another source of inspiration was Laplanche (1992) who offered a philosophical dimension in thinking of transference as being the psychoanalytical situation. To identify the other within oneself on a profound level and at the same time contain the enigma of the analysand: "Yes, you can take me for an Other, because I am not what I think I am; because I respect and maintain the other in me" (p. 246). This view opens to think about the transference as something always ongoing and profound, like a geography rather than a phenomenon. It captures a poetic and cultural dimension in relation to the transference, and how it can appear within and outside the psychoanalytical context. Psychoanalysis doesn't exclusively belong to the consulting room, but to the world.

I ask myself, where on or along the described river I localize myself now? Well, I do have a boat, and I have a map to navigate from initially given from you but onto which I continue to draw. I notice a psychic presence beginning to feel like a psychoanalyst which differs from being a psychoanalytically oriented psychotherapist. The distinction is subtle yet clear. Not being a full member means still being kind of an outsider and nevertheless I clearly belong. The psychoanalytical world lays more open than before.

Dear Institute, thank you for your engagement and for providing space, time and depth for the psychoanalytical legacy. I feel grateful, rich and proud to be a part of it.

Regards from a candidate in progress,

— Eva Christina Tillberg

# 10  A letter to the Czech Psychoanalytic Society, Prague, Czech Republic (1936)

## Jakub Kuchař

*Our psychoanalytic society is rather small (around 35 members and 35 candidates) and very much influenced by the history of our country which was occupied twice during the 20th century. We had to spend more then 40 years under the rule of communistic totalitarian regime. Czech psychoanalytical community survived these unhappy times of our history in the "underground", only because of a small number of psychoanalysts, to whom we are grateful to these days. After the Velvet Revolution, Czech Psychoanalytical Society could gradually be officially reestablished.*

*The current training requirements for graduation in the Czech Psychoanalytic Society are:*

- *completing minimally 600 sessions of your own training analysis (minimal frequency is four-times a week),*
- *after the first year of your training analysis you can start to attend lectures if they are to be open (new cycle of lectures, in our institute, usually start every third year),*
- *completing four years of lectures (90 minutes every week or 180 minutes every other week),*
- *pass the exam on psychoanalytic theory,*
- *writing a theoretical paper related to one of the lectures and defending this paper in front of the panel of training analysts,*
- *when you finish two years of lectures, you can start your first control case,*
- *finishings two control cases (minimally 300 sessions each, minimal frequency four times a week) under supervision (minimally 75 supervisions for each case),*
- *writing a case study for one of these cases and defend this study in front of a panel of training analysts.*

*I am describing current situation (December 2022). New president of our society and the team around him want to make substantial changes in our training system.*

—

DOI: 10.4324/9781003465409-10

Dear Institute,

There were moments when I hated you. I hated your rigidity, I hated your subtle totalitarian tendencies, I hated your hypocrite pretending that our training is flawless and that problems are only in us candidates with unresolved Oedipal issues! I know that my anger really came from my unresolved Oedipal issues. But I think it is very easy to stay with this level of explanation and downplay your impact on the given situations.

When I first found out what psychoanalysis really is, I fell in love with it. I was amazed by depths within which psychoanalysis understood the complexities of inner life of individual human beings. When I started my training in our institute, I tended to idealize experienced psychoanalysts. I wanted to know what kind of people they are, I was curious about their personal lives. I thought that they are very special kind of wise and mature people. After some time, I found out that it is not always so and that quite often they are just normal human beings with their narcissistic tendencies and flaws. Of course, finding out some of these things made me angry.

One of the most popular concepts in Czech psychoanalysis is the totalitarian object. And it is not a coincidence. During the previous regime, a lot of Czech people had to hide their true attitude towards the outward socio-political situation and were forced to follow wishes of those who were hierarchically above them. And such a constellation inevitably leads to the epidemic of totalitarian objects among people. And not only epidemic of people around, but also an epidemic among us, members of psychoanalytic community. It is obvious that by studying totalitarian objects we also try to deal with ourselves.

Furthermore, I think, dear Institute, that our psychoanalytical society (and therefore also we candidates), to these days, is still influenced by somewhat conflictual relationship of the psychoanalysts who helped our psychoanalytic community to survive during the previous regime. Their attitude towards psychoanalysts was rather different. I think that historical trenches from this period of our history are still here. However, I think that similar phenomena could be probably found in almost all communities which share some history. And recently, the conflicts in our psychoanalytic society became more explicit and we started to discuss them. And I think it is much better than behaving like that there are not any.

To be concrete, one of the things, I personally found annoying about my training was that quite often its conditions were not clear, explicit and unified. Candidates and people interested in our psychoanalytic training, if they wanted to have a clearer piece of information, had to wait on the decision of training analysts. For instance, first years of my training, you could find on our webpage contradictory pieces of information about requirements for applicants for training in our institute. On one part of our website, you could find a piece of information stating that our training is also open for professionals from non-clinical setting, on different part of our website, it was stated that this training is only for licensed clinical psychologists and psychiatrists. Or it was very annoying to find out after about 4–5 years of my personal psychoanalysis, when we were finally allowed to start out control cases, that it is strongly recommend continuing personal analysis during our first control case. As someone who was not well-off and had to really calculate every penny to be able to pay for his training analysis, I would like to know these things in advance to be able to reckon on them. I also did not like how strictly some lecturers of our institute differently (and quite often contradictory) defined what psychoanalysis is and what psychoanalysis is not. I understand that different psychoanalysts have a different opinion about the essence of psychoanalysis. However, in my opinion, I think they should be aware that their colleagues from institute may have a bit different opinion and sometimes not to present their personal view of psychoanalysis so confidently and one-sidedly (at times even dogmatically).

Dear Institute, I don't want to be only critical. There were many great parts of our training, for instance theoretical seminars. These encounters with more experienced psychoanalysts were a great experience which enriched me clinically and intellectually. It helped me better to connect abstract theoretical psychoanalytic ideas with concrete psychoanalytic clinical work. We also created a great cohort of candidates. We could discuss our perspectives on psychoanalysis with each other and by these discussions we could consolidate these perspectives more deeply. The important part of these seminars also was, of course, meeting later for a beer and discuss everything regarding our institute informally! At this time, we created bonds that will most likely last till end of our lives.

I am also happy that you gave me an opportunity to participate in the organization Fenichel's Prague Conferences. I could get to know more international psychoanalytic environment which was a great experience for me. At similar time, I also started to participate in the European IPSO events which were very enriching as well. I am always amazed how it is easy to create connections with people who have passion from psychoanalysis, even if they come from very different backgrounds.

It is difficult for me to talk about the experience of my own analyses. My first analysts died after four years of my training, and I had to start second analysis with another analyst. I think I still really cannot acknowledge the death of my first analyst. (Thank you for your handling this situation, Dear Institute. A few hours after it happened, one of the members of the training committee called me and empathically told me the sad news. Another of your members, in the coming weeks, gained access to my psychoanalyst's materials and officially confirmed the number of sessions I underwent. And my soon-to-be new training psychoanalyst did her best to quickly found the capacity in her practice.)

Today, I see both of my analyses very enriching but at the same time very different. It is interesting to see how psychoanalysts, who were also good friends, work psychoanalytically differently and, for instance, tend to interpret very different phenomena. It made me to be more aware of how diverse psychoanalysis really is.

Some time ago, my current analyst used a word "family" when she talked about our psychoanalytic society. And this word stuck in my mind, Dear Institute. There are many historical grievances in our society. There are many things which makes me angry. But there is also a strong affect which connect us. We share a strong passion for psychoanalysis. We also share some history and identity. And, I find to be part of my growing up to be able to better tolerate imperfections and narcissistic tendencies of the leading members of our institute without becoming too "paranoid-schizoid" very quickly and activating my own inner totalitarian objects. It also helps me more easily accept my own (moral) imperfections. And these days, new president of our psychoanalytic society and the team of people around him want to change our institute to make it more egalitarian. I am hopeful about these changes.

— Jakub Kuchař

# 11 A letter to the Italian Psychoanalytic Society, Rome (1936)

*Valentina Palvarini*

*I am a candidate at the National Training Institute of the Italian Psychoanalytic Society, SPI, which was founded in 1925 and officially recognized by IPA in 1936. SPI is the largest of the two IPA Societies in Italy—the smaller one split from SPI in 1992. The National Training Institute is divided into four training sections—two in Roma, one in Milano and one in Bologna-Padova (my local section)—and adopts the Eitingon training model.*

*I am a former IPSO representative of my section and a current IPSO member, as all Italian candidates are (our Society pays for our memberships every year). I share my training path with a class of six other colleagues and a few dozen candidates in my local section. In the whole National Training Institute there are about 200 candidates. We are a heterogeneous group of professionals of different ages (however, one can apply for admission to the Institute only up to 45 years old) and diverse backgrounds (psychiatric, psychotherapeutic, psychological and educational previous work and trainings). This makes intergenerational dialogue and exchange among different levels of experience and backgrounds a special characteristic of the relationships among candidates, not just of those among candidates and graduate and training analysts.*

*We attend a four-year program of seminars. At the end of every year, in order to pass to the following year, the candidate has to discuss a short clinical-theoretical presentation with two training analysts. To access the final graduation exam, one must have completed all seminars and two control-case psychoanalyses, followed under weekly supervisions for at least two years each. With the IPA Board approval for variation of the Eitingon Model in recent years, control cases and training analyses can now be conducted at 3–5 times a week.*

*I'm a psychologist and before becoming a candidate I have had a previous training in infant and young observation and work with young people and families (Tavistock method). I now work privately with adults as well as with children, adolescents and parents. In the past, I worked as a nursery teacher. I believe this experience, together with my observational studies, has been a fundamental step between my university studies and the beginning of my clinical work as a psychoanalyst in training: it allowed me to dive into the*

DOI: 10.4324/9781003465409-11

*sensory-bodily experiences of the first phases of life, a treasure for my present and future clinical work.*

—

Dear Institute, Dear Analysts, Dear Analysts in Training,

Starting to write this letter was not easy. I procrastinated, held back by the resistance to expose myself personally as a candidate/analyst in training. Then, I started writing at the last minute, I guess to privilege spontaneity, not letting myself have the time to subject the text to repeated chisels and sweetenings. Basically, I would like to offer my thoughts and feelings with the passion that I would have in front of a real and trusted interlocutor, in a situation of open dialogue and understanding. I could have skipped these difficulties behind the scenes and have presented the finished product. Instead, I want to talk about this conflict about feeling free to express openly as a candidate because I believe it is a very frequent and key experience among candidates. I would also say it is a normal experience among students, but I think it has some peculiar features and consequences among us, future analysts, that need to be deeply investigated, not only at one's personal analysis level, but also at an institutional level. Certainly, this experience takes different forms in each one, but it seems to me that it often might extinguish the enthusiasm for participation.

Of course, as highlighted in *Dear Candidate* (Busch, 2020), times have changed and nowadays the climate of dialogue between psychoanalytic institutions, training analysts and candidates is so much more open and conciliatory. Probably, a few decades ago, this book itself would not even have been thought of. I can imagine that the maturational process of psychoanalysis and psychoanalytical Institutes over the last century laid the ground for me to write this letter.

While in many occasions we are encouraged to participate and express freely, I am also sure that often, inside a candidate's heart, questions like "will this opinion put me in a difficult position in my Institute?", "should I expose myself in front of training analysts that one day might be my evaluators?", "have I really thought deeply enough about this and made it interpretation-proof before talking about it?" frequently prevent candidates from getting involved more actively in discussions and institutional participation. There may be various reasons for this of course, from neurotic fears to reasonable concrete worries, but looking at the whole, it seems to me that the group/institutional aspect of the matter really deserves more attention (and sounds fascinating to me).

Here is a quite common example. In my local section, a seminar about institutional consultations with subsequent referrals to other clinicians was recently held. Many interesting things were said and discussed, but many just remained concealed in the mind of some candidates. When the seminar was over, I heard whispering: "but at the end of it all, what is the point of having consultations conducted by some clinicians to later refer patients to other therapists?". I felt some important chance to discuss freely had been lost in the seminar, beyond what one could think on the specific subject. Why didn't this candidate feel safe enough to express this basic question? Why wouldn't an average candidate offer his/her candid doubt in a scientific discussion? My point is that it seems to me that precisely basic questions, those that challenge what lies at the foundation of subjects and is often given for granted, are often still felt as too uncomfortable to discuss. Instead, I think that posing just these questions, simple but not banal, would give the opportunity to our teachers to offer their best pieces of knowledge, and, to us, to keep alive the amazement of the child inside ourselves, during our training.

As for me, when I was invited to participate in the project of this book, I wondered what contribution the thoughts of one candidate among many, and a quite young one, could add. I still had in mind the letters full of wisdom and kindness from great analysts around the world collected in *Dear Candidate*. I answered myself by reversing the question: why should there be a particular justification, a special title, to accept with gratitude and fearlessly the invitation to be present and active? So here I am, driven by the desire to actively participate in my psychoanalytic training, in the hope of seeing my "psychoanalytic siblings" doing the same, each in their own way, and having the opportunity to continue learning from them too.

Earlier, I called myself a candidate/analyst in training. The fact that in the psychoanalytic world, there exist these two ways of calling students, which convey different shades of meaning, makes me think. It seems to me that the expression "analyst in training" rightly recognizes the candidate's desire and daily passionate attempt to think and work analytically. In part, perhaps being called "analysts in training" also involves a narcissistic identity gratification that makes one feel like the "grown-ups" when one is still "small". But these grown-up/small, mature/immature dichotomies do not exhaust the complexity of reality and this suggests that the process should be rather looked at. To me, thinking analytically basically means thinking freely. This ability certainly takes a long, long time to develop, but when the candidate begins control cases in supervision, I see him/her as the seed that already contains much of the information and nutrients that will make up the seedling, even if water, sun and nutrients of the earth will be needed as well. Especially, and this is perhaps the aspect that I perceive most powerfully, the expression "analyst in training" recognizes the candidate's position of effective analytical responsibility towards his/her patients. "Candidate", on the other hand, alludes more to the student's desire to become part of a community. Dear Institute, while this aspect is natural and necessary, I feel I am training to be a person who learns from the community to use psychoanalysis to care/cure, not to be a psychoanalyst among psychoanalysts opposed to non-psychoanalysts (and this is a very strong siren song for all of us). Much has been said about the infantilization of candidates. The way I feel as a candidate is perhaps closer to an adolescent position, if we follow the metaphor of the ages of life. That is when idealizations and identifications are put to the test of experience in the world. In our case it is a matter of diving oneself in the clinical, scientific and institutional psychoanalytic reality while creating one's own personal way of doing it. I also realize that I am speaking as a candidate in her thirties not having many years of clinical practice behind her. Maybe some colleagues in their forties or fifties would not feel in the same position. It is also this diversity of personal experiences that makes us such a rich community.

Of course, I am not interested in being called a candidate or a student or an analyst in training when I perceive sincere welcome and respect from my teachers. For example, it happens to hear psychoanalysts of the highest caliber calling candidates "colleagues". Each time I find it moving and this makes me feel accompanied with regenerating trust towards a profession in which a lot of trust is needed.

It is the sense of freedom and the consequent responsibility that psychoanalysis give me, that are stronger than the fear of exposing myself, that push me to participate in this book, to be involved in IPSO activities, to ask questions during seminars, to seek exchange. With psychoanalysis, I have learned that speaking aloud with someone else about one's personal experiences, in appropriate spaces, times and ways, usually expands the depth and truth of internal and external dialogue. I can be wrong, I can change my idea or reinforce it, but the important thing is to elaborate it with others.

Dear Institute, speaking of dialogue, I often think of the multiplicity of psychoanalytic models and particularly on how they communicate with each other or not (actually, how analysts communicate with each other or not!). It's a theme that crosses many letters in *Dear Candidate* and that I feel it crosses our Italian training too. Although in Italy we probably don't have such profound differences in theoretical orientations as there may be found in other countries, I sometimes wonder how much the experience of training in another section, having different theoretically oriented teachers and supervisors, a somewhat different cultural-historical background, would actually change my learning and practice. I am talking mainly about different clinical-technical orientations: how does a Freudian work? How does a post-Bionian work? And an object relations-oriented psychoanalyst? Moreover, does what we think of a clinical method correspond to the clinical practice of each analyst? It doesn't seem that having grown in a specific theoretical tradition necessarily results in a strictly corresponding clinical method. This sounds like a synonym of maturity, where learning has not been applied mechanically to clinical practice, but it has gone through a process of adjustment in the personality of the analyst. What happens in the middle between didactics and clinical practice is what I am interested in. While, of course, coherent and solid references are needed, I feel that while building my own way of becoming a psychoanalyst I get nourishment when I can source a wide range of possibilities of identification and experience. In our Institute, we have these opportunities. For instance, I know I can attend to conferences organized by other sections or ask for supervision to analysts of different orientations. I would greatly appreciate if these possibilities were provided by the Institute as an integrated part of our training. It's true that every section has its own peculiarities due to history and cultural context and this is something to value. However, I think this wouldn't be conflicting with the creation of more spaces to compare models and clinical methods and have our teachers really compare their points of view. This could be really enriching and clarifying about what usually is passed down through whispering "between the desks" and can feed the sense of belonging but not scientific debate.

Likewise, the critical sense and the curiosity for humans that led me to undertake this training, urges me to take a few curious gazes not only towards different models of psychoanalysis, but also towards other disciplines, such as neuroscience, which are equally concerned with the human being. Some years ago, the National Institute organized a conference with a famous Italian neuroscientist, that was attended by all candidates of all the Italian sections. That day and through the following years I have heard quite polarized opinions on that conference (and it was just a conference, not a whole training program!). Some candidates felt enthusiastic about the message from the Institute about welcoming neurosciences. Some others firmly disagreed on what they considered to be, if not devaluing, at least trivial for our training. Dear Institute, this wide division makes me think we still have a lot to do to get off our sacred psychoanalytic ivory tower.

One could argue that learning to be a psychoanalyst already requires an enormous commitment and that thinking of opening up to extra learning during training could waste energies. It could also be interpreted as a defense against fully immersing oneself in one's experience. In fact, I am not interested in fast accumulation of knowledge about other models or disciplines but in perceiving, and this already happens many times, that my teachers and my institution value diversity and encourage questioning and comparison, as the scientific method suggests. When, albeit rarely, the famous categorical expression "this is not psychoanalysis", said or meant, peeps out, my sense of wonder and curiosity are mortified. Clearly not everything can fit, but I wish I could hear more frequently "Is this psychoanalysis? . . . What is psychoanalysis? . . . How can we help this patient using a psychoanalytic mind in this context?". I appreciate that we have come a long way over the last decades, however I would like to posit that we still have some miles to go to traverse the distance from authority to sincere curiosity. Usually, I have the impression that on occasions in which such a sharp vision is presented, the discussion dies down and bystanders end up silently divided between those who agree and those who disagree. So comes the end of a constructive dialogue. Of course, these are inherent dynamics in the very variety of people and institutions. We can learn this way too if we approach it without too many idealizations.

I remember a teacher once said that "theories are metaphors". I feel it is precisely the openness and dialogue between different theories and sciences that allow us not to reify them, not to fall into the trap of matching the symbol with what it represents, but rather to find the invariants, beyond the specific dialects. Sometimes and with a lot of working through, this might even allow the reciprocal fertilization of different disciplines with their respective knowledge. As another teacher provocatively said, of course not meaning to push us to laxity, but to taste experience: "don't read psychoanalysis books, read the great books of literature!".

Dear Institute, my personal analysis and my training so far taught me that the experiences from which you really learn are the ones done together with the Other: with your analyst, with your supervisors, with your colleagues . . . and with the group, the famous fourth pillar of psychoanalytic training. I learnt that grouping means bringing together plurality and diversity, in others and in ourselves, but it can also mean avoiding these things when the impact is too destabilizing. Staying and working in a group involves an important narcissistic challenge, it confronts you with your own limitation and partiality, but it also helps to better recognize your riches to share.

I am now thinking of different types of groups: the group of different theoretical models and different psychoanalytic communities around the world, the group as a device for clinical work and thought, the group as a human condition for growth, etc. Dear Institute, especially when I have the opportunity to fully experience a group dimension, the knowledge I have assimilated individually or in a two people setting, as in supervision, starts to resonate with other pieces of learning inside myself, comparing, conflicting and hopefully, one day, finding some integration. I feel my internal orchestra needs continuous rehearsals and attunements between instruments before playing the concert. In the same way, learning in and through the group can allow to learn better to meet differences, use them to enliven the experience, tolerate them or, at least, represent them.

The international candidate organization, IPSO, is a good group in which it is possible to broaden one's theoretical, clinical, cultural perspectives and is an expression of candidates' desire and ability to participate. I feel this is an important complement to my local training: occasionally breathing winds that come from afar allows me to oxygenate the air in my environment and to relativize the difficulties I encounter there. Dear Institute, I am grateful for the collaboration with IPSO representatives during these years. In general, taking part to international events, such as those organized by IPSO and IPA (very much facilitated by online meetings, as in the case of IPA webinars and IPSO "Meet the Analyst" events), makes me feel a member of a large world community where creativity sprouts up from shared passion for psychoanalytic thinking and idealizations can be reduced among the variegated possibilities. But as I feel I am aware of this breadth of international opportunities, I am not sure it is perceived by all. I wonder why. Is it just about the difficulty of speaking and understanding English? Is it because candidates are already very busy with their local training? Or does this also have something to do with a training culture still quite rooted in bi-personal settings? In international containers of this kind, differences are valued and similarities raise feelings of understanding and sharing. However, I believe, it is when we are confronted with the colleagues who are close to us that the convergences and divergences, put in tension by physical and cultural contiguity, become more incisive and fruitful. For this reason, dear Institute, I would greatly appreciate if the group, as a fundamental dimension of experience, was increasingly implemented in the structure of the training. I wish there could be more of seminars on group theories, experiential groups, group supervisions, spaces for discussion on training experiences, study of institutional dynamics and meetings between candidates from different years and different local sections.

Institutional dynamics is the last topic I would like to pose and also the one that somehow encompasses the previous reflections. Dear Institute, I perceive that many resistances lurk in the great container of the institution, and generally this is not a subject of discussion. The same fear I spoke about at the beginning of the letter, which dissolved while writing and was replaced by the pleasure of thinking and imagining future meetings, is, yes, in part, the expression of my personality tendencies, but to the extent that these encounter institutional dynamics. We know everyone has a peculiar way of articulating one's own characteristics with the fantasies and experiences that concern the group and the institution. However, not everything can be exhausted by "analyzing the matter with one's analyst". Something must also be analyzed at other levels. There is a whole world of discourses around institutional dynamics that flow like streams of water underneath the cities. These can simply emerge to the surface, when the ground is compact and openings are left free, or they can erode the subsoil and cause collapses. I believe it is a common experience that many of the issues regarding the institutional level are only discussed in personal analyses, whispered in supervisions, shared with colleagues who are most trusted, in short, in informal and intimate circumstances. Nothing is strange about this, but it is a background with a considerable influence on the life of an institution. So why not extend the field of psychoanalytic observation to the institution, for example, to the dynamics of power, to how institutional transference and countertransference influence training and the professional life after? Certainly, I'm not talking about publicly exposing private issues, I'm thinking about fully recognizing the institutional dimension of Training as a container whose very processes influence contents and learning. What I was imagining above about a greater implementation of the group dimension, in seminars and experiences, might go in this direction.

My question was once answered: "You can't peek into your parents' room". Instead, I believe that the door of the parents' room can never be completely closed, nor can this be expected, precisely because even the best institutions and the most seasoned analysts are simply human and immersed in the same game. Furthermore, this answer suggests that "everything happens just in there", in the mythological rooms of the Training Committees, when instead, if it is an institution we are dealing with, we are talking about the role and the link between all its members. I come back here to think about the active participation of candidates in their training. When dialogue is led keeping in mind the characteristics of group and institutional functioning, the communication of the individual is considered more as an element emerging from the group than something as a clue of a personal conflict. It seems to me that usually, in this environment, people feel reassured and more willingly offer their thoughts as resources.

Finally, dear Institute, dear teachers and dear fellows, there would still be so many aspects of my training that I would love to share and discuss. However, the issues presented above are basically the ones that remain most open in my mind, the kind of questions that cannot be easily answered and need to be extensively shared. This is one of the most important life lessons I have absorbed with psychoanalysis: never stop asking questions to oneself and others, never stop nurturing your ability to grow.

For everything else, I really look forward to meeting you, dear teachers, dear colleagues, dear travel companions.

—Valentina Palvarini

# 12 A letter to the Argentine Psychoanalytic Association, Buenos Aires (1942)

*Natacha Julia Delgado*

*The Argentine Psychoanalytic Association was created on December 15, 1942. At the Argentine Psychoanalytic Association (APA) the tripod training model corresponds to the one proposed by Eitingon: didactic analysis, didactic supervision and training seminars. In 1974, the curriculum at APA was modified and curricular and academic freedom was voted for. The spirit of this reform was rooted on a proposal that encouraged a singular training design in combination with an institutional plan. Having in mind the idea of implementing an analytical pluralism, the plan was that each student-candidate would manage their training and freely organize in what order they would want to approach different subjects at the pace that seemed most convenient: "that each one could have access to the teachers and the types of thought that most interested him or her, so that study would maintain or regain its legitimate share of pleasure instead of being a subduing demand" (Baranger, 2003). This was based on the idea that each candidate could build*

an itinerary according to his previous knowledge, his current interests, his future plans and the eventual vicissitudes of his real life (for example, availability of time in a certain period, pregnancy, illness, etc.). But this freedom in the choice and order of the subjects and in the rhythm of their completion is framed within very concrete parameters; at least twelve courses (half of the curriculum) must be of study and deepening of Sigmund Freud's work; one must write two papers, a theoretical research text about an analytic concept and a monograph on topics dealt with in seminars to present them and hold a discussion with fellow students and professors

(Aslan, 1980)

—

Dear Institute,

The desire to start the training program at the Argentine Psychoanalytic Association was an effect of analysis. Different transference currents intervened.

DOI: 10.4324/9781003465409-12

A couple of years before formally taking that decision, I had started a master's degree program in psychoanalysis, which was the first occasion that APA dictated a post-graduate academic program jointly with a private university. I must say that although the academic experience had its ups and downs, one of the most important facts for me at the time was getting to know as teachers several APA training analysts. These analysts had a different style of questioning and reading psychoanalytic texts— especially Freud's— that pleasantly surprised and intrigued me.

My analyst at that time was a graduated member, however the indication of the Institute was that before authorizing my full admission I had to undergo an analysis with a training member, at least for one year. The regulations required me to make this change. At that time, I considered that complying with this demand made sense although I had mixed feelings about changing analysts. I suppose I understood that this move— hypothetically— implied good functioning and institutional organization.

Later on, I had the chance to re-think about the matter. After reading Kernberg's list in his famous article "Thirty methods to destroy the creativity of psychoanalytic candidates" (1996), who—with fine irony—states that it was necessary to slow down the processing of candidates' applications, to postpone their admission; to delay the provision of information in order to help candidates become slow and ineffective, I wondered about my case. I should say that the delay in admission, apart from what Kernberg points out, had another deleterious effect, of which I became aware sometime later: it somehow facilitated a process of idealization with respect to the institution, its functioning and its members. I believe that my desire to join in and the postponement, based on the compliance of a rule, convinced me—partially—about the rigor and seriousness of the institution. Regarding idealization, Tomasel (2016) referred that

> Calich et al. (1995) understand psychoanalytic training as a process of identity formation and see idealization as a motivational force and also as a defense against the anxieties aroused during training. They describe the deviations of the idealization process, which can, in some cases, lead to excessive idealizations. They warn that the institution and the analysts should function as guarantors of a normal process of idealization, since, if the process of de-idealization of the analysts who participated in our training and theories evolves favorably, there is an acceptance of the limitations of the idealized object, which recovers its real aspects.

Over the years, fortunately, the process of idealization suffered its vicissitudes and without falling into the opposite effect of disillusionment and disappointment, I was able to establish a less regressive, more realistic and also more personal relationship with the Institution.

As you might well know, the ability to experience an institutional climate of freedom is key to work through different issues without fear of retaliation.

I enjoyed learning and participating in activities and seminars, while endur-ing different kind of transferences. Nonetheless, I think when it comes to options for seminars, it may be worth it to offer other kind of topics. I agree with what Freud proposes in his dialogue with an impartial person in the text "The question of lay analysis (1926) when he says:

> If—which may sound fantastic today—one had to found a college of psychoanalysis, much would have to be taught in it which is also taught by the medical faculty: alongside of depth-psychology, which would always remain the principal subject, there would be an introduction to biology; as much as possible of the science of sexual life, and a familiar-ity with the symptomatology of psychiatry. But, on the other hand, ana-lytic instruction would include branches of knowledge that are remote from medicine and which the doctor does not come across in his prac-tice: the history of civilization, mythology, the psychology of religion and science of literature. Unless he is well at home in these subjects, and analyst can make nothing of a large amount of his material.

In addition, I would add an introductory course about the history of each local institution. The implementation of this course could be a useful starting point for any training institute.

My intent here is far from sounding preachy or like I am giving you—my dear Institute—a piece of advice. However, another key point that I realized it might be worth informing candidates at the beginning of their training are the research and reading tools available at APA. For example, the fact that the library holds more than 30,000 available copies (books and journals) of psychoanalytic bib-liography (it can be seen reflected in the database that the library has more than 150,000 bibliographic references, including books, chapters and articles of journals of our discipline). The digital access to its official publication, the APA journal, that gives the chance to an expanded vision on diverse topics and authors at both local and international levels. The degree of importance given by you in your training program would profit when being in turned with the idea of pluralism acknowledged also by the fact that APA happens to be an Institution member of the International Psychoanalytical Association.

I highlight these points, dear Institute, because I find that a wide array of psychoanalytic authors may become great traveling training companions, in the sense that they are interlocutors for clinical work, colleagues who have thought and written about topics that may interest us and with whom we can share vicissitudes and doubts regarding our clinical practice. Getting acquainted with different authors is also necessary to prevent us from falling into a state of self-induced "blindness and deafness" and also reflect upon our supervision, seminars and personal analysis experiences.

I would like to think that you, dear Institute might find interesting what Jacobs (1994) pointed out—referring to a candidate in training—about another important subject:

Having experienced little understanding and effective <u>interpretation</u> of his own nonverbal communications in analysis, and having been exposed to little teaching about the subject in supervision or in courses on technique, he can be expected neither to appreciate the importance of the nonverbal dimension in analysis nor to develop competence in working with it. The result, all too often, is that in his clinical work the candidate uses his ears to the virtual exclusion of his eyes, focuses single-mindedly on the verbal material, and sooner or later develops a scotoma for material expressed in bodily language or through other nonverbal means. In this way a significant deficiency in <u>analytic technique</u> is transmitted from one generation of analysts to the next.

I would also like to express that the participation of candidates in different levels of the institution, and also in scientific exchanges both nationally and internationally, should be enthusiastically promoted. Obviously, each path is unique, and to promote does not mean to enforce. In my case, the experience of participating in different committees (psychoanalysis and culture, permanent training, library committee, history department) made it possible not only to meet with other colleagues and exchange ideas, but also to understand the functioning of my own institution. The nature of integration and joint activities with members of the association means that the Institute does not function in isolation or separated from the rest of the institution. Otherwise, one can say that one of the negative aspects that can arise is the risk of infantilization of the candidates. I smile as I recall the countless times my peers in training and myself were referred by older members—all training analysts—as "the kids". An ambiguous compliment when one happens to be over forty years old.

The wonderful part about being a candidate, dear Institute, are the numerous paths that open before us. For example, several years ago I became part of a peer supervision group with colleagues from other IPA training institutes—with other mother tongues and other psychoanalytic cultures—that allowed me not only to listen to the reading of clinical vignettes in unknown languages, but also to deal with a difficulty that, in turn, we were able to transform into an instrument of clinical and theoretical reflections. This circumstance, that is, the different possible ways of listening to a clinical presentation through a group work, gave me, for example, the chance to get more acquainted with the illusive and complex concept of reverie, among other things.

Apart from that, one of the activities I enjoyed the most, came after having participated in the European Congress for Candidates in Paris where I presented a paper jointly with Dr. Marcos de Soldati (APA candidate). After that, I spent one week in London in October 2017, visiting the British Psychoanalytical Society and Institute as part of IPSO's Visiting Candidate Program.

It is also worth sharing here some other thoughts about training, in this case, by Zac (2002) who pointed out some years ago:

it is necessary to take into account the particular characteristics of each institution. Although in the beginning there was only one psychoanalytic institution, today they are scattered in all continents, and although there are common criteria with which we identify ourselves as analysts, there are cultural and socioeconomic differences that give us our own existence. That is why we must think more and more about including new openings to the community and the academic world, while considering the complexities in giving continuity and durability to psychoanalytic theory and its practice.

My intention here was to express some ideas based on my own journey but also to reflect upon my bond with you dear Institute. Understanding the history and functioning of one's institution, the complexity of the training model one is on and the fact that our views might change along the way, are key to a successful analytic training. Analytic training aims at a singularity in the development of an analytical identity, and for this, it seems important to appreciate the multiplicity of paths that are there for one to take. It also implies that the training does not stop at formalities established by institutional regulations.

Sharing my experience and suggestions has been one of the many possibilities I could think of when writing you this letter. I am sure there are others. As Bolognini (2008) reminds us that "the different transfers during the analytic training path are with supervisors, with classmates, with the institution, with the authors, with colleagues who are analyzed with the same analyst, with the analyst's own analyst", etc., . . . and all of them are part of the training experience. Yet, this might be a topic to be addressed more in depth in another letter.

I must go now. Hope you enjoy the reading!

— Natacha Julia Delgado

## 13 A letter to the Institute of Psychoanalysis of the Chilean Psychoanalytic Association, Santiago (1949)

*Gabriel Rivera Constanzo*

*The Institute of Psychoanalysis of the Chilean Psychoanalytic Association (APCh) has been authorized by the IPA to train psychoanalysts since 1949, together with the acceptance of the association as a component society. Dr. Ignacio Matte Blanco was the founder of the APCh, which in its beginnings was marked by contact with the British Psychoanalytic Society, where Matte Blanco did his psychoanalytic training. In the beginning, Matte Blanco was a didactic analyst, teacher and supervisor, whose functions converged in the same person, generating transferential conflicts. With the training of psycho-analysts, this situation changed through various reforms. In the 60s, conflicts arose between psychoanalysts of the APCh, mainly between some who were interested in integrating psychoanalysis with psychiatry and universities and another group who wanted to keep an independent development. Between this decade and the 70s, an important number of members emigrated, among them Otto Kernberg (to the USA) and Ignacio Matte Blanco (to Rome). This was also a time when socio-political (military dictatorship) and economic factors hindered the development of psychoanalysis in Chile.*

*Gradually, the candidates have been able to participate in the scientific activities of the Association, which in the beginning was not possible. Also, with time, the curriculum of the training was extended towards the French current. Currently, the training has been extended to another region of the country (Concepcion) allowing to diversify the psychoanalytic training in our country.*

—

Dear Institute:

I am writing these words at an advanced stage of my psychoanalytic training, I have already completed the theoretical seminars, I have completed my two official supervisions and I am currently in the process of preparing my two final monographic papers to become a member of the Chilean Psychoanalytic Association (APCh). I look back and it seems that time has passed very quickly, that 2017 when I started the training seems to be there, very close, but

DOI: 10.4324/9781003465409-13

five years have passed that have been convulsive. It was my turn to go through the institute from crisis to crisis, first an institutional crisis that resulted in a division of the psychoanalytic association, then the biggest socio-political crisis in recent history in Chile and, in a kind of overlap, the global health crisis resulting from the COVID-19 pandemic, which transformed psychoanalytic training into a virtual format for a while.

My relationship with the Institute goes back several years, perhaps about ten, when the idea of doing psychoanalytic training at the APCh, which was the only IPA institution in my country, began to circulate in my mind. But I was constantly hearing about an elitist, conservative and rigid institution. Those same points made me doubt about joining, until I got closer to different activities, met psychoanalysts of the institution and I realized that everything that was said had more to do with certain prejudices than with reality. It took me several years of thinking about it until I decided to apply.

I remember the happiness I felt when I received the information that I had been accepted at the institute. It was a year before starting the theoretical seminars, and I immediately contacted who I wanted to be my analyst, because, at that time, there was a certain number of didactic analysts to whom the candidates had to have access. Who I had in mind to start my analysis had only one place available, fortunately I was able to take it, otherwise I would have had to start my analysis with whoever was available on the list, rather than by choice. Currently it is no longer that way, but there is an increase in the number of analysts with the possibility of fulfilling the function of didactic analyst, this function has been extended to members with the status of full member.

I remember that the week before starting the theoretical seminars the IPA World Congress of Psychoanalysis took place in Buenos Aires. I had the opportunity to attend with a group of five classmates. From that moment, an affectionate and precious bond was born between us, which I value very greatly, which allowed us to sustain a training that, as I mentioned at the beginning, went from crisis to crisis. For me it was very stimulating to participate in that congress, as I was able to glimpse something of the psychoanalytic movement within the IPA, besides meeting and sharing with fellow candidates from different parts of the world, which made me value even more the decision to carry out my training as a psychoanalyst in the IPA.

However, at the same time, we learned that there were strong conflicts within the association between groups of associate members, who were resigning with the intention of forming a new association, which finally came to fruition. This situation was difficult for me and my colleagues. It was a time of great uncertainty, of not knowing what would happen to the institution and, therefore, to our training. Fortunately, those who directed the institute made us part of the situation that was being experienced, we were invited to days of reflection, and we were openly informed of the possibilities that were to come and the care that would be taken with us as analysts in training. It was reassuring to be included, in some way, in the context that the association was going through. These were difficult moments that we were able to overcome together.

The beginning of the theoretical seminars was very stimulating and, at the same time, demanding for me. Hours and hours of study made me value the training at the institute. We studied in depth Freud, Klein, Bion, Winnicott and Lacan, who were the authors with exclusive seminars for their work. I am not going to describe the whole curriculum, although it was a very complete organization of seminars. Except for seminars dealing with psychoanalytic work in and with the community. I highly value the quality, the theoretical and clinical level of the teachers I had during my training. I never felt a doctrinal and dogmatic style, as I heard people say before I joined. In general, there was a concern for each analyst in training to find his own style and his own voice psychoanalytically speaking. I especially noticed this in the official supervisions I had. This is a point for which I am very grateful.

Just as we were emerging from the institutional schism that had occurred, a socio-political revolt took place in Chile as a result of unsatisfied social demands accumulated over many years. It was in October 2019. There were daily demonstrations with many people in the streets, among which pockets of violence were generated. I lived in the vicinity of where the largest demonstrations were taking place, and I was an eyewitness to the situation on the streets. A great majority of people demonstrating peacefully, with artistic demonstrations, musicians, dance, different performances; and also, a minority of people who produced violent outbreaks that the media showed more frequently. There were fires, looting, destruction that were less generalized than what the media showed. Police repression was brutal, with situations of human rights violations, with more than 8000 victims of state violence, more than 400 people with serious eye trauma due to pellets, about 30 dead. The situation was very serious. At the institute there were some days of reflection on the matter, and a public statement was published; but it seemed to me, personally, a reaction not so forceful for the gravity of what was happening in the country.

The days of protests went on day after day, for months. Until the COVID-19 pandemic arrived. The training changed to a virtual format, care, supervision, seminars, personal analysis, the tripod was established online. Social uncertainty began to transform into health uncertainty, the situation was delicate worldwide. The institute tried to safeguard the training within the possibilities offered by the context. There was support for the candidates, for example, in reducing the fees for didactic analysis and official supervisions during the period when the economic situation was more fragile. We will still have time to determine what will change in psychoanalytic transmission as a result of the changes produced in the pandemic period. For me, I think it was possible to continue the theoretical seminars without major inconvenience, as well as the supervisions, where I felt that I valued the presence more was with my personal analysis and my control analyses. Fortunately, I was able to return to the different training activities before the end of the cycle.

During my training period I became involved in institutional politics through the candidates' organizations. First, I was the representative of my group to IPSO and OCAL. These experiences opened up a whole world outside my institute. I began to meet candidates from other countries and other regions, which was very important, given that my institute is small and dialogue with foreign colleagues was something very vitalizing for my experience. Through IPSO I had the possibility of doing a "Visiting Candidate Program", where I visited the Institute of Psychoanalysis of Barcelona, which was a very enriching experience for my training. I attended seminars and supervisions in a different environment than the one I was used to. I noticed some differences in how training was organized in a different region. This possibility was very stimulating.

In addition, I had the opportunity to participate in the board of directors of OCAL, where I was able to share the work with a wonderful group of colleagues, colleagues from Mexico, Panama, Nicaragua, Venezuela, Brazil, Argentina, Paraguay and Chile, we formed a phenomenal working group. My role was from the scientific secretariat. In part, my experience of the visit to the Barcelona institute gave the possibility of devising some kind of similar experience among the candidates from Latin America, and so the board generated an institutional exchange project, where a candidate could participate in seminars and supervisions in an institute of another country in the region, this to take advantage of the virtual format resulting from the pandemic. It was a project that was highly valued by those who were able to participate. My experience in OCAL was very gratifying, especially in generating links and ties with colleagues from different countries, which has been called the "fourth leg" of the tripod. I think it has been an additional enrichment to the training at my institute. So much so that I am still part of the board of OCAL, now as vice-president.

Also through OCAL, I have the possibility of representing the Latin American candidates in the Commission of Formation and Transmission of Psychoanalysis of FEPAL. It has been an invaluable experience in my training. A Commission that has wanted to give voice to Latin American candidates and invited one of us to be an integral part of it, and where I have had the opportunity to work together with Latin American analysts of vast experience and generosity. I have also had the opportunity to speak at different international meetings in order to raise and open dialogues on the training experiences of my peers and colleagues. At the meeting of institutes organized by the commission, I had the opportunity to have a dialogue with Adriana Prengler, who was then vice-president of IPA, where we were able to talk kindly and frankly about the points of training that I present in this paper.

The training period is very stimulating, challenging, incorporating psychoanalytic thinking is fascinating, especially when we begin to notice the transformations that take place in our lives. It is also a demanding period that brings pressures and discomforts with it. One of the constant concerns in my institute and the various institutes in Latin America is related to the high economic cost of training in institutions linked to IPA. It is a recurrent and transversal issue, which is tangentially made explicit because it seems to be an issue of bad taste, but we know that it is always there as a backdrop. This generates a kind of elitization in the access to our training, which also imposes a barrier to entry, since many applicants to our institutions give up as soon as they learn about the high economic cost involved. We are left with those who, in one way or another, can assume these costs, which generally refers to a specific group of the population with a certain economic level, which establishes a kind of social endogamy. I think this is a problem in our institutions, in relation to inclusion and diversity issues. It is often said that psychoanalysis is in crisis, that there are few aspirants to be trained, of a kind of relegation before other therapeutic approaches more effective, more in line with the pressing times and it may be, although it is also seen that Psychoanalysis arouses great interest in general, in university students, in different media, in social networks, in open seminars, in the circulation of psychoanalytic literature, that is to say, there is a lot of psychoanalysis circulating outside our institutions. So, what seems to drive away many potential people to enter the institutes is that same elitization, which is homologated to a kind of conservatism, which gives an impression of a psychoanalysis in crisis, but that seems to be a problem of our institutions.

Dear Institute – our training *is* elitist, no doubt, but does it have to be so?

Many of us, before entering the training, have developed our working life in contexts of social vulnerability, in public hospitals, in public health systems, in the community, but we have had to abandon those places to prioritize work in private practices that will make us earn a better income to pay precisely for the training. We are closing ourselves up in our practices and working with people who can pay our fees, which are also increasing. The community, in its different aspects, imposes itself on us, but we have done our training in a sort of bubble; in most institutes there are no seminars dealing with psychoanalytic work in and with the community. We move away and we do not know how to get back. For example, in general we do not participate in the elaboration of public policies.

Our Latin America is so diverse, so multicultural, but if there is something that makes us very similar is that we live with social, economic and political crises permanently. In our countries inequality, social vulnerability, poverty, discrimination, racism abound. Psychoanalysis has something to say, of course it does. Although our specificity as analysts is the unconscious in its multiple manifestations, we are not anthropologists, or sociologists or political scientists, and from our specificity we have to dialogue with other disciplines and knowledge, but beyond academicism. It is not sustainable to be ostracized. Psychoanalysis has to be involved in the socio-political processes of our peoples, from our specificity, but it has something to say in the unrestricted respect for human rights, in the defense of democracy as a social organization, in violence, in racism. These are issues that have been distant and distant in my institute in the course of training, and I think they are very necessary to address. I am inclined and advocate for an inclusive psychoanalysis that, from our specificity, is inserted in the socio-cultural and historical processes that permeate the context in which it unfolds; it is necessary to leave the offices themselves and, as a specialized resource, generate efforts to get closer to the different needs of mental health in society.

Finally, I would like to say that I feel a deep gratitude for these years of training; they have been arduous years of growth and very stimulating. I am grateful for the formative process and the possibilities that have opened up for me within the Institute and also outside, which I have tried to take advantage of. I thank my colleagues, my teachers, my analyst, my supervisors and all those who develop their work in the APCh, also those who make up the candidate organizations such as IPSO, OCAL and ABC, which have been a nest of friendships that will last for the rest of my life. I thank my family and friends for their company throughout this period. Becoming a psychoanalyst is a path that never ends and I embrace it with passion thanks, precisely, to this training.

(Dedicated to my father, who I lost in 2023)

— Gabriel Rivera Constanzo

# 14 A letter to the Japan Psychoanalytic Society, Tokyo (1955)

## Naoe Okamura

*Editor's note: Instead of including a brief history of the Japan Psychoanalytic Society (JPS) at the outset, the author has woven it into his letter.*
*The requirements for graduation from Japan Psychoanalytical Society are:*

- *Attending lectures*
- *Two control cases, more than four times per week, longer than two years, under once a week, in-person supervision by training analyst*
- *The completion of your own personal psychoanalysis by training analyst*

—

Dear Institute,

A senior psychoanalyst once told me, "I don't encourage you to apply to the Institute. There's nothing good about joining the Training Institute in Japan." To me, this is an enigma embedded in my relationship with the Institute. It is something that I have thought about these years and would like to explore on the occasion of writing this letter.

The advice was from a highly intelligent psychoanalyst with experience at a prestigious organization in Europe. He took his time and kindly advised me. I cannot recall his words precisely, but I understood that he was saying that compared to his experience abroad, where psychoanalysis was authentically taught and practiced, psychoanalysis in Japan was not genuine. He suggested that I consider applying to a training organization abroad, and said, "What I told you is a fact, and it is up to you whether you proceed with the application."

As time passed, something heavy started to take root in my mind. What would all these years of training be for if it were a sham? What about the psychoanalysis I have been undertaking already for years? If what I have been undertaking were not psychoanalysis, what is the definition of psychoanalysis? I wondered if I did not understand all these because I was surrounded by con artists. If that were the case, there could be an environment somewhere in which I would feel confident that I was experiencing true psychoanalysis, a condition akin to a golden womb. Then I'd better go abroad. The analyst

DOI: 10.4324/9781003465409-14

who gave me advice was so confident because he had experienced that golden environment in Europe. But then why did he choose to come back? How is it possible to take part in an important organizational position in the Institute in Japan yet recognize that the training is not worth taking? These doubts could have been poisonous. I lived with them in the hope I could metabolize them.

I am sincerely grateful to the analyst, who shared his honest views and ultimately assisted me with my application to the Institute of JPS. Still, it remained as an enigma that I could not solve. My puzzlement was partly because I had predicted the opposite. A few years earlier, when I first expressed my wish to join the Institute to another training analyst, his expression turned grim. He said sternly, "A psychoanalyst-in-training should be someone who has gained a certain high reputation in the field of psychoanalytic therapy. Only those with the requisite skills and personality should be allowed to apply. You are not there yet." I apologized for my thoughtlessness but said that I thought I was allowed to apply because the application is for training, and through the process of training, I may be qualified or fail. He replied that only the most promising can receive training because resources are limited. This was true. I knew that there were only four training analysts at the time in Tokyo, a city of 14 million people. I understood the situation, but his words created the impression that the Institute was an exclusive, referral-based membership club. Although there were other opinions that mildly encouraged me to apply to the Institute, the vehemently opposing views on the Institute greatly affected me.

Life training at the Institute was neither exclusively privileged nor futile. The first new thing I experienced was attending the monthly meetings of the Tokyo branch of the Training Institute of JPS and the series of seminars hosted by the Institute. At the monthly meetings, case studies were discussed in a variety of terms by members with real ease and openness. It was an atmosphere of enjoyment. At first, I was nervous to attend these discussions, but I gradually came to enjoy them. Regarding my personal analysis, it went on as it had been, as I had started years before. What changed was that I now had a chance to happen to be with the analyst. Of course, we avoided encounters, though there were inevitable circumstances like Institute meetings, which remained as stimulants in various ways on the couch. I often made remarks that I longed for the time I could keep utterly distant from my analyst. I must say joining the institute made some sessions stormy, and I cannot more than appreciate how the analyst maintained every session with a steady, insightful, and fostering attitude. The most difficult and time-consuming task was to find a patient for psychoanalysis. The word psychoanalysis remains unfamiliar to the public in Japan. Many candidates need to find patients with unconscious needs and the capacity to benefit from psychoanalysis and introduce them to control cases while fostering their motivation by increasing insight in psychotherapy. This is a difficult task for somebody who had never done the psychoanalysis before.

The enigma mentioned earlier re-emerged in my mind when I had a chance to learn about the history of psychoanalysis in Japan. Psychoanalytic concepts appeared in the psychological journals in Japan as early as 1912, and Yabe Yaekichi became the first Japanese IPA member in 1931. Though no group was able to maintain substantial and consistent activity during World War II. In 1955, psychiatrists who were interested in psychoanalysis gathered under Heisaku Kosawa. Kosawa, who undertook psychoanalysis from Richard Sterba in Vienna, had privately conducted clinical practice with psychoanalytic ideas before and during the War. His activities led to the foundation of the Japan Psychoanalytical Association (JPA) in 1955 with Kosawa as its central figure. At the time of its establishment, the JPA absorbed some of the functions of the IPA Japan branch. Later it separated and while the JPA continued its activities to introduce psychoanalytic ideas to a larger group of clinicians, the Japan Psychoanalytic Society (JPS) resumed its activities as IPA Component Society.

The following problematic facts were revealed by the whistleblower to IPA in early 90s; JPS had practiced "psychoanalysis" as low-frequency psychotherapy (up to twice a week). After the on-site investigation, followed by years of generous support, guidance, and assessments by IPA, the JPS reestablished the regulations and bylaws to meet the IPA requirements for training, which came into effect in 1996. Since the issue was notified to JPS at the 38th IPA congress held in Amsterdam, it became called as the "Amsterdam Shock." It had a tremendous impact on candidates at the Institute at that time. For them, it was not merely an update for proper psychoanalysis. In 1993, the JPS Institute had 87 trainees which was reduced to six after the reformation. They needed to change their career plans to conduct psychoanalysis. Some may have felt deceived and betrayed by the leaders of "psychoanalysis." I wonder how the members, especially the training analysts, felt about the incident.

Reformation took three years, and efforts were made by both the JPS and IPA. The extremely frequent meetings of the JPS Steering Committee and the Consulting Committee on Japan set up by the IPA helped the JPS develop. Still, the biggest effort must have been made after the new regulations were applied. Under the new rules, the training analysts who used to conduct "psychoanalysis" as psychotherapy once or twice a week now needed to practice psychoanalysis four or five times a week with candidates. Although many had experience of psychodynamic and psychotherapeutic training abroad, the quality and quantity of each experience varied, and few were qualified as psychoanalysts at Institutes abroad. I would not be surprised if their practice were a series of trials. The struggles and hardships of the training analysts at the time are entirely understandable, while it is hard to assume how they were feeling about the situation. Did they think they were heroes for bravely confronting calamity, or did they follow obediently and remain unconvinced? Did they unconsciously feel shame? I would state those training analysts were the pioneers of Japanese psychoanalysis in a somewhat embarrassing situation in the 90s. Many of those leading "psychoanalysts" of Japan remained in leadership positions in the JPA, an organization mainly for psychoanalytic psychotherapy, while within the JPS, where they struggled with the unfamiliar proper psychoanalysis, which they themselves had not undergone. In this unique situation, they gained their clinical experience and contemplation of psychoanalysis.

At the same time, this aspect became the main reason why some Japanese psychoanalysts claim that the practice in Japan is no good. Those unhappy with the current situation of the Institute may be challenging the IPA's guiding policy at that time when analysts without proper training remained training analysts' status. They might resent how legitimate psychoanalysis had not been handed down to them in an honorable tradition. I have heard the following condescending comments several times from different members: "They have changed the regulations passively just because of external pressure." Perhaps it is based on the value that individuals are independent and should not be easily shaken by others. However, it is how we Japanese live in society, dealing with pressure comes from the something present externally, both as individuals and as a state. These pioneers, and the history of psychoanalysis in Japan, remind me of a pattern recognized in Japanese history, especially in relation to more powerful foreign countries.

Approximately 80 years ago, after Japan became a challenger to the international community, it brought tremendous suffering to neighboring countries, and was defeated. The new authority, the occupant forces, arrived from the overseas. Some Japanese felt deeply betrayed by the Japanese leaders who misled them totally. Some identified themselves with the leaders and committed suicide. Meanwhile, some felt silently guilty for survival. Led by the occupant forces from the United States, modern capitalism and democracy were at once introduced. Reformation continued, and we absorbed much from abroad and rapidly became an industrial nation.

We can see a similar pattern 200 years ago, when the isolation of the Edo period ended, and the arrival of foreign ships, most notably American black ships, forced the opening of Japan to the outside world. This event made the government of the time look small to the Japanese, as they recognized that something stronger existed far away. Japanese intellectuals traveled to the West and hastily brought back advanced knowledge and systems, which contributed to the modernization of Japan. Thus, the repeated relationship with something unknown and powerful came from afar and was always crucial for significant change.

This pattern is not limited to the modern era. For more than 2,000 years, Japan has been dependent on the neighboring empire of China for culture and technology. In ancient times, Japanese had no characters to inscribe our own language; we had no organized social structure for govern the nation. It was China who introduced us to the characters, urban design, Buddhism, and Confucianism.

Thus, for us Japanese the advanced has always arrived from overseas, and our own indigenous culture is not formal. The difference between attributes of the import and the domestic could remain distant after years. This can be seen in Japanese classic notation system. The native spoken language was not considered official, and for Japanese, the formal written language was in Classical Chinese. Even today, academic books are written in high-sound Japanese with frequent use of Chinese Characters, including Freud's translations. Kitayama, who promoted the clinical study of the Japanese language, discusses the psychic duality of the Japanese. The duality between the formal imported Chinese characters and the vernacular spoken language could be related to the psychic duality. Depending on other advanced countries lead to various group sentiments. The admired and advanced place, where the ideal object stays, is far away, separated by the ocean. We are always an aggregate floating on the edge of relationships, and we maintain our identity by trying our best to absorb and not be swallowed whole. The history and geography of Japan might be related to the theoretical attention to the relationships associated to dependence, such as the Ajase complex and Amae.

I might have written too much about history and culture. Having written this far, I realize this may not be a situation unique to Japan. If there is a particular advanced central region, there are peripheral area. Something similar in Japan could happen in other countries. If we consider the individual and not just the country or Institute, we can say that we all have a marginal nature, for we have all been babies born into the midst of all that is advanced. We human beings, once infantile, all have some marginality within.

I recently stumbled upon an article in which the analyst mentioned at the beginning of this letter stated that when he himself applied to the Institute, he was told by a senior analyst that there was "no meaning in joining."

Dear institute – Is this to be a traditional rite of passage in the JPS? Could this be an intergenerational transmission of conflictual expression? Can nothing be done to address this repetition compulsion!

What advice would I like to offer the younger clinician considering pursuing psychoanalytic training? As I am convinced that undertaking training at this Institute is not meaningless, I could tell the next generation that they can expect genuine experience at the Institute in Japan. At the same time, there is an alternative to undertaking training abroad. Psychoanalysts trained at other institutions or in foreign countries will continue to be valuable to our community in Japan. Since psychoanalytic practice and theory are deeply rooted in the West, it is always worthwhile to study in a Western culture. There are also great differences in schools, techniques, training systems, and social environments, and I feel that having people with different experiences is essential for a small Training Institute. I have learned and will continue to learn from both analysts who have trained abroad and those who have not. I believe that a group of people with different backgrounds and values can enrich a group, as long as we can recover open mind from time to time, accepting our marginal identity.

I cannot end my letter without mentioning my own Institute experience. The Institute is a training institute, but even if I were to complete each training item individually, it would be completely different from the experience of belonging to the Institute. An institute is where people are born, grow up, move in and out, and disappear amidst a constant gathering of members, which is like a home. The members are akin to siblings who share the same parents. Each has its own personality and clinical practice style, and they continue to practice psychoanalysis in the shared climate of Japanese culture. Each member stimulates me and opens parts of myself that I did not know existed. In that sense, the Institute is itself a complete environment in which to learn psychoanalysis. What is happening in the environment is intertwined with my analysis, the experience of patients, readings, and case discussions.

Finally, I want to mention IPSO, the candidate connection worldwide. I have already written about how Japan has relied on the outside world. Thanks to the development of telecommunication tools and frequent online "meet-ups," as seen during the COVID-19 pandemic, I have been feeling IPSO colleagues closer than ever. To me, this fellowship feels different from that of the Institute fellowship. If the Institute's fellow candidates are my brothers and sisters at home, the IPSO candidates worldwide are the people I meet when I open the door to my house and venture out into the city. There is a great deal of freedom, and something new always makes you look back, understand, and develop an original version of what you have experienced at home.

Dear Institute, I would like to express my genuine appreciation for belonging to you. To transmit the experience of psychoanalysis, there should be a group of people willing to devote themselves to it. I hope to pass the pure joy and value of being part of the psychoanalytic community to the next generation.

— Naoe Okamura

# 15 A letter to Asociación Psicoanalítica del Uruguay, Montevideo (1961)

*Ximena Palabé*

*The Institute to which I belong is part of the only Association in my country, a small country with a little more than three million inhabitants, which has the largest concentration of population in its capital, and as is commonly said, a country in which we all know each other. The Association celebrates almost 70 years of its foundation and is governed by the Uruguayan Model approved by the International Psychoanalytical Association (IPA), character- ized by groups of didactic functions.*

*Training at the Institute is based on three basic pillars: individual analy- sis, seminars, and supervised practice. The analyst conducting the individual analysis may not intervene in any of the institutional decisions concerning the analyst in training, including admission to the Institute, which is in the charge of the Admissions Committee.*

*There are no didactic analysts but analysts in didactic functions, which can be all Associate Members after a certain time of entry as a member.*

- *Currently, it is a requirement to pass 18 semester seminars once a week, which are freely chosen among the proposals offered each year by the group of Full Professors, having to comply with a certain number of semi- nars by areas. The design of the curriculum allows us to mix between dif- ferent generations in an intergenerational conformation.*
- *In the first four seminars, a brief written work is carried out in each one as a note, and then a written production per year must be presented in a seminar of choice during the following three years. The notes and papers are discussed and commented on within each seminar where they are pre- sented, and the approval of the work and the seminar is independent. The exchange and questioning of the classmates who have been in the Institute for years, as well as the Titular and Adjunct Professors who lead them, give an extremely enriching vision and look.*
- *The maximum number of years to complete the 18 seminars is six, and ten years to complete the training.*
- *Supervised practice requires a minimum of two supervised analyses for at least two years, which must be approved by each supervisor.*

DOI: 10.4324/9781003465409-15

- *The analyst in training must present and get approved by a "Commented Session", which consists of a session of one of the supervised analysis processes with comments and reflections, along with a transcript of the session without comments. This written material is presented to a Commission of the Senate of Supervisors composed of two analysts who evaluate it.*
- *Once all the requirements mentioned above have been met and approved, a final written work with theoretical-clinical articulation must be submitted, which is the work that enables the passage to Associate Member.*

*The Association has important national and international recognition and provides solid theoretical training, possibly the main reasons that arouse interest in admission. It propitiates in the collective imagination something elite, of privilege for those who enter, and of a select group, replete with fantasies present both inside and outside the Association.*

—

## Transiting the endless formation

Dear Institute,

When I thought about writing about my experience of the journey through training as a psychoanalyst at the Institute, I remembered a situation where, in the privacy of the office, in a first meeting with a psychoanalyst, someone said: "Where to start? That's so many things!" The psychoanalyst sets out to listen to what emerges in an attempt at evenly floating attention, encouraging free, abstinent association in a quest to give rise to suffering.

For me, case-by-case research, theory, and clinical work are inseparable in psychoanalysis. Theory helps, supports, and offers possible lines to be thought along so that the dyad may tolerate something of the enigma and uncertainty which is always present in our work with our patients.

It is difficult to pinpoint when my interest in psychology and psychoanalysis began. Readings in adolescence, experiences studying theater at that stage, and approaches to reading Freud in high school possibly knotted and aroused curiosity about psychic suffering, together with one's own sufferings. I began to study psychology, I discovered psychoanalysis in college, I began to analyze myself, novel in my family in which I am not preceded by university or professional students, and where psychology and psychoanalysis were nothing close or known from any point of view.

I began my first analysis while studying for my college degree with an analyst who had no institutional affiliation, which at that time did not worry me. I already graduated with a Bachelor of Psychology, with greater knowledge of institutes and associations linked to psychoanalytic psychotherapy and psychoanalysis; present institutional transfers led me to a second analysis, an analyst with broad institutional membership that would allow me to choose where to present myself. I think that, at that time, there was already the desire to train as a psychoanalyst at APU, the only Association belonging to IPA in my small country.

Years, events, growth, and various professional and personal changes passed, until sometime later, I began a third analysis with the idea and desire to present my aspiration to join the APU Institute. As usual, I had two admission interviews, the minimum required established, and my application was accepted.

It is not naïve or accidental to choose training in Institutes within Associations and Societies that belong to IPA. I wonder how much influences the search for recognition, valuation, and wanting to belong to a group that is not freely accessible, in which you have to be chosen and accepted. Or perhaps obtaining a degree that consolidates a habilitation is still illusory because the internal and proper qualification of being a psychoanalyst is what really legitimizes it.

Dear Institute, I share some reflections on my transit through your enclosure, hoping to resonate in the agreement or the discrepancies, and it will no longer be my thought only but of everyone in which they echo.

I thank you that, from your operation, the participation of analysts in training in institutional instances is promoted and enabled. People in the group elect representatives to the committees; we are listened to and valued in a true integration, exchanging horizontally, without the hierarchies being made noticeably enforced.

My experience is that this institutional participation does not protect us from locating ourselves and being placed in infantilized places. Rhythms, loves, and hatreds unfold, as in so many other areas from which we are not alien. It is proper to our condition as human beings, of the instituted and the instituting, with all that it entails.

Within the Association, the places and functions of analysts and analysts-in-training are clearly delimited, but it is not so clear to the outside. The analysts in training are not members of the Association as long as the formal requirements are not met and the vote is made for the Assembly General; meanwhile, for the outside, "we are all APU".

I wonder how much this process conditions us to institutional belonging – a belonging designed forever. Breaks, ruptures, and individual disengagements that precede us account for strong movements, which, perhaps in our psychoanalytic institutions, due to the imprint of transfers and idealizations, acquire another tenor with the implication of institutional membership agreements and disagreements.

Upon entry, after receiving your acceptance letter, I was greeted by fellow analysts in training with a warm welcome, a traditional meeting that we usually do every year. It has become a kind of ritual that welcomes, contains, generates belonging, summons, and calls for participation. I tend to get intensely involved, so from the beginning, I responded to that call. From the first year, I actively participated in institutional work from different insertions.

I consider that it makes belonging and commitment a way of being; I do not conceive another way of getting involved (although I understand and respect that each one has its way of participation, its rhythms, its times, and its choices). This comes at an expense because of the exposure it requires. When you question, disagree, and participate actively, you are offered criticism but also recognition, which is what we yearn for.

What we call the fourth leg of the tripod, which refers to the meetings and exchanges between analysts in training and institutional life, acts as support, accompanies us to make the path less lonely, and helps us overcome the obstacles we encounter during the journey. I embraced and clung to its importance, surely in a search for reassuring shelter from the busy beginnings. I think that sharing, exchange, and filiation are fundamental parts of what makes us approach associations.

Thanks to these institutional insertions, I was able to link and connect with colleagues from all over Latin America and the world in a close exchange bond.

These experiences, as well as participating in conferences, congresses, inter-institute group supervision, allow me to get out of the inbreeding of your corridors and the Association, endogamy fostered by being a small group. Movements of idealizations and de-idealizations are essential processes to enrich training and promote growth.

Exercising the role of representative of the group of analysts in training led me to question myself about the function of such. It is an arduous and difficult task; at the same time, it becomes rewarding, formative. We must not lose sight of the fact that it is a transitory, temporary place, and we must bear in mind that the organization is the one that transcends. It is essential to prioritize the interests of the organization and the majority of its members over personal ones. To be a spokesperson, defend and sustain these interests, and position oneself from what is considered valid, valuable, and beneficial for those who integrate them because organizations are made by all of us who belong to them. The learning and the bonds of affection and friendship that are generated are invaluable gains. We share a passion for psychoanalysis, a work sustained in incompleteness and not knowing, an uncomfortable place, which moves us to a permanent questioning, in personal analysis, the main leg of the tripod.

The task of being representative, being part of a board of directors, left an indelible mark on me that transformed me and will always accompany me.

I think it is difficult to raise questions and discrepancies with your functioning, even more so from the place of an analyst in training. Pending the approval of formal instances that will be evaluated, there is excessive care to what to say; it is avoided to participate so as not to be located in a place of possible ally or enemy of certain thoughts, theories, or groups, which exist within the Association. Persecutory aspects are reactivated.

I assume that some of these experiences are present even after being Members – affiliations, protagonisms, where to be located or not to be located – and it seems that most of the time, it matters more who is speaking than what they are saying.

Dear Institute, I think we should problematize these aspects more openly, which often hinder institutional and collective life.

Evaluation is a controversial topic in our specificity. Much has been written about transference in psychoanalysis and much has been exchanged and discussed on these points in Congresses.

My questioning is based on the fact that there are as many different evaluation criteria as there are analysts exercising teaching function, integrating a commission of evaluation of *Sesión Comentada*, of work of passage to *Miembro Associated*.

It enriches this difference of criteria and of styles, but at the same time, it generates confusion because certain parameters that unify are not clearly established.

Dear Institute – would it be possible for you to establish them?

I understand this task would put us at a crossroads because establishing these criteria would lead to a rigidity contrary to our specificity, which restricts, but at the same time, seems to be necessary to make it enriching and orderly or reassuring for those of us who are being evaluated. In addition, there arises the question of whether it is even possible to evaluate a task that focuses on the singularity of each case. There is always so much that is not visible within the analytical field, and what is shown is always just a slice the unconscious in the transferential heat is, in some aspect, inaccessible.

Several experiences of our own generated discomfort, bitterness, and a response that was not expected. Perhaps it is difficult for us to accept something of the failure of ourselves, narcissistic ideals of perfection, superego mandates, and, like children, we want total approval and make parents-analysts-teachers proud – a complex dialectic that is installed in the interplay between evaluated and evaluator, leading to a reactivation of children's aspects.

Do we allow ourselves to disagree, debate, and freely question our supervisors? I wonder if it has to do with idealization, with transferences, with the fantasy of being expelled or rejected, and if there is room then for an intergenerational exchange from a position that enriches without other readings that obstruct. Because, sometimes when there is disagreement, an exchange of back and forth is not always installed but used to exercise a place of power and supposed knowledge by those who are evaluators.

It is a controversial point when analysts-in-training are put in the position of young apprentices when, most of the time, we are professionals in the third, fourth, or fifth decade of life, with years of trajectory and experience. The "young people" of the Association are almost grandparents, an interesting paradox.

The idea is to encourage one's own thinking, but to what extent? 'One's own thinking' could lead to a work or a commented session that is not approved! It is a difficult task to produce new experiences without being trapped in models that officiate as dogmas.

Works read by supervisors, teachers, and colleagues from whom we receive praise are harshly criticized and disapproved by others, and these discrepancies are not always processed without leaving wounds, a point we are told should be more worked in depth in our analysis and reanalysis.

The discussion about high or low frequency is recurrent, and the borders and edges seem diffuse whether it is psychoanalytic psychotherapy or psychoanalysis, whether we can think that psychoanalysis is all that a psychoanalyst should practice, whether it is defined by analytical listening or only by the high frequency and the use of the couch . . . how far is it possible to diversify and make our praxis more flexible without losing what identifies it as psychoanalytic?

Dear Institute – we candidates recognize the changes of the time in sexuality and in family configurations. I ask of you – are you training us to receive each one who comes to our offices with their particularities, with their demands, and with their texts and subtexts typical of this time?

It is challenging enough to find enough openness to include these topics within the training in the seminars without running away from the analytical function without thinking about the times we receive these patients! Such issues tend to generate controversies, and such insertions are devalued most of the time. They deserve to be thought about in depth.

We are crossed by the vertiginous in terms of the immediacy of information, the eruption of social networks, and the advance of technology. It challenges me to think about how psychoanalysts are adapting and integrating it into our praxis. But, it feels as if fundamentally, with regard to the adaptation and modification of our organizations, such changes are resisted by the institute.

Dear Institute – I ask that you also include in your seminars how to develop a psychoanalytic identity beyond the Association – outside the office, in the interdisciplinary, and in the community. Continue and preserve the legacy left to us by our predecessors, along with a desire to add others, without feeling that we betray this legacy. Build from the path already traced, of successes and errors, without ignoring the history that precedes and constitutes and conditions us.

We are summoned as the future of psychoanalysis, but ambivalences prevail!

In relation to the curricular supervision that you demand of us, I think about how much it interferes with the work of analysis and how concerned we are that that patient does not abandon or interrupt the treatment. We tend to show and talk very little about treatments that fail, both analysts and analysts in training. Dear Institute – we owe ourselves more fruitful and open exchanges on these topics in formation.

I think that each of us must sustain our practice from the singular, with its own style, and we must ensure that theories, institutions, and especially institutional transference does not inoculate us against growth.

I thank you, my dear Institute, for the differences you encourage me to continue questioning – forming myself without deforming or formatting myself. Situations that make us uncomfortable, that lead us to disagree, undoubtedly make us grow, similar to what happens with our patients – such discomfort is necessary.

Analytical thinking carries the particularity of each analyst that is put into play in each analysis, in each unique transference situation. The relativity of knowledge is inherent to analytical positioning. It is an extremely laborious task for us, this training to become psychoanalysts, to be able to tolerate the swings of internal and external anchors while a psychoanalytic identity is permanently strengthened and built. De-idealizing you – the Association – and the theories in order to bring ourselves closer to our own creative thoughts is so necessary in our task of tolerating not knowing, uncertainty, and castration.

The trick is to strengthen our identity as psychoanalysts so that it continues to be questioned throughout our trajectory and clinical practice because, simply put, we will always continue to train.

— Ximena Palabé

# 16 A letter to the Psychoanalytic Society of Porto Alegre, Brazil (1963)

*Rafael Mondrzak*

The Psychoanalytic Society of Porto Alegre (SPPA) was founded in 1963 in the city of Porto Alegre, in the state of Rio Grande do Sul, Brazil. Affiliated to the International Psychoanalytic Association (IPA), it is well known nationally and internationally, with members actively participating in the presidency, board, and several committees of the IPA, FEPAL, and the Brazilian Psychoanalytic Federation (FEBRAPSI).

SPPA's Institute of Psychoanalysis (IP) has years of experience in offering the path of psychoanalytic training. Currently, to begin the process, the candidate must be in analysis with a full member of the society for at least one year before beginning the theoretical seminars. These seminars have a duration of four years. In addition, 200 hours of supervision with two different supervisors with two different cases are required, with the patient attending at least three times a week. To become an associate member, the candidate must, after completing all these initial steps, present a clinical paper demonstrating his or her analytic work to the teaching committee.

The IP also includes the Candidates Association (AC), an internal organ of the institute where candidates and analysts dialogue constantly and openly about training, the paths of psychoanalysis, as well as promoting high-level scientific events.

Predominantly Kleinian in its origins, SPPA has, with the passage of time, come to count on the growing presence of French and North American post-Kleinian authors. The fundamental axis of the training is the chronological study of Freud's work.

The interest in Kleinian ideas was brought from Argentina by Mário Martins, Zaira Martins, and Cyro Martins. Celestino Prunes, even though he trained with a classical analyst in Rio de Janeiro, also exerted a great influence in this sense. There was also a great influence of the Kleinian developments through the work of Hanna Segal, Bion, Meltzer, Winnicott, etc.

In the early days of the Society, we had the presence of Kleinian analysts through the interchange with Arnaldo Rascowsky, Leon Grinberg, Willy Baranger, and Horácio Etchegoyen.

DOI: 10.4324/9781003465409-16

*We have also received, throughout the years, exponents of psychoanalytic thought such as: Leon Grinberg, Betty Joseph, Ruth Malcolm, Elizabeth Spillius, Christopher Bollas, Stefano Bolognini, and Antonino Ferro among many others.*

*From the beginning, developments in the psychology of the Ego were also incorporated into the teaching curriculum, through the works of Hartmann, Kris, Loewenstein and Margaret Mahler.*

*The Society's contact with the French school was increased with the visits of André Green to São Paulo in 1976 and Porto Alegre in 1994; Janine Chasseguet-Smirgel and Bela Grunberger in 1978 and 1987; René Diatkine in 1981.*

*Since 2005 the study of the authors of the French school and the intersubjectivity current—the space in scientific thought of Baranger's concept of analytical field—have become an official part of the training curriculum at the Institute of Psychoanalysis, including also original texts by Lacan.*

*In general, the basic line of work in our society has been oriented towards the valorization of the clinical fact, always taking into consideration man's biological roots with its instinctive vicissitudes and primitive object relations as the determining model for the development of psychic reality. As a link between these two poles, we emphasize the concept of unconscious fantasy.*

*The consequence of this conceptualization for our clinical practice has been, independently of individual theoretical positions, to reaffirm the importance of maintaining the setting, the method of free association, the use of interpretation and reconstruction in the systematic and early analysis of transference neurosis and the use of counter transference.*

—

Dear Institute,

I am glad that I was able to stop to write you this letter. Time seems to run faster than we want it to. But I have learned from you the value of communication, so I think it can beat time, if we allow it to. And let's face it, we both know that a letter is never just a letter. What that letter means, we must wonder. But I don't want us to start like this, worried about the motivation. Just as I don't want to write it in fear of what you might think of it! It seems that the more we combat our neuroses and ambivalences the more they appear. My letter will be about my thoughts and insecurities of our trajectory and . . . . great. That's life and this letter has to be the way it is.

When I first contacted with you, you already existed in my head, in a platonic way, but you were there. Your first speech was strong, firm, and with imposing tones: *"if you really want to get into a relationship with me, you have to have at least one year of analysis at least four times a week".* I thought at the time that it excited me to wait, even though I felt anger, because I was already under analysis three times a week, and now, I was receiving a command that in my fantasy represented that I was a more problematic person. I want you to know that I am trying to describe my feelings of that time, but I am constantly invaded by mine of today and I find that precious. Regarding our first contact, today I am eternally grateful that you offered me that one year of elaborations. During this period, I was able to take you from heaven to hell, from perfect to imperfect, from idealization to reality. I am sorry if only today I can recognize this. I don't blame you directly for that initial seesaw ganging up. You were being yourself, and I, childishly (unfortunately), was being myself. I needed this polarized mechanism as a way to organize and elaborate my own ambivalences: good versus evil. You, as an institute that trains psychoanalysts had to be a God and then the devil. God in all its perfection, an institute that holds all knowledge—provider of the Bionian "O" if you may, and soon after, imperfect for not fulfilling my initial idealizations. Fortunately, I have discovered with time that the seesaws of life, when they have on each side realistic weights, tend towards a harmonious balance, even though they preserve the differences between each part. In other words, you could naturally be above me, like an organizing establishment. I just did not need to heroically place you so far above or so far below in a villainous position. It was vital to our relationship, that I could realize this functioning, initially through this abrupt oscillation of the seesaw, and then capture the gentle winds that brought me what would be the reality of our relationship.

After this first stage was over, the other requirements for finally entering into a serious relationship were already metabolized. I would have to talk to three colleagues so that you would get to know me better, and I could then begin my first four years by your side. How exciting this first moment was. Intense meetings, watered with much reading, I discovered how much you enjoyed reading Freud, but also Bion, Winnicott, and Klein. You showed me a new world and I felt I was dating someone with a lot of experience. Meltzer, Civitarese, Ferro! Oh, how much we had to talk about all of them! You have a much more open mind than I even imagined! In addition, you offered me multiple possibilities to immerse myself in your psychoanalytic world, with scientific activities, congresses, and conferences. If I could describe it, I would say it was my enlightenment time and how grateful I am for it. I don't know if at any other time in my life I will experience a learning curve as intense as the one you offered me among so many professors and seminars. As a bonus I gained classmates, dear colleagues, and relived the exciting adrenaline of school life.

With my good behavior, at the end of the first year, I won from you the right to put the couch in my office, along with the authorization to take my first case for analysis under your supervision. It was with the couch in my office that I felt your physical presence. When I looked at that couch, eager to receive inner worlds, I knew I would be with a piece of you forever.

Honestly, I think your willingness to walk me through the first 200 hours of my new couch was crucial. Just like learning to ride a bike, you used to say that nobody goes out riding alone and that it can be dangerous! I no longer felt that I was receiving orders, but rather guidance. I was scared to analyze a patient and going under supervision was a sigh of relief. I knew that those two hundred hours were going to be our longest commitment, beyond our seminars. It was an arduous commitment, with rules and fears to be able to maintain an analysis. Although with a small feeling of plastering, I quickly understood that these two hundred hours fortified the theoretical background of the seminars. You were trusting in my abilities. I was riding a bicycle with two small children supporting wheels, with you running beside me.

This was our most intense period, we met in seminars, in supervisions, in our scientific activities, and eventually I had to talk about our relationship in analysis. I admit that I felt a weariness and many times I was tired of you, but I took a deep breath and went back to routine: seminars, supervision, and analysis. I remember that you always talked about this tripod that would ground my training, with the importance of providing me with a solid foundation. I agree that there is no other way to relate well, if we don't have this tripod well established, which not only sediments knowledge and maturation, but also allows you to see further and more stably the path to becoming an analyst. As I mentioned, during the periods when I was tired of you and took a deep breath, I learned that the "analyst profession" would demand a similar tolerance from me. Often tiring, thankless, and other times relaxing and extremely beneficial to me and the patient. I think that I will forever go through critical moments with my patients and even with psychoanalysis that will demand long breaths.

It was after four years, I had one of the small-sided wheels removed from my bicycle. I should no longer meet with you to study together. That was the end of the seminars. I complained so much about the fatigue of what you asked me to read from one week to the next . . . funny, it was also from one week to the next that I began to miss you for the first time. My first encounter with the fear of losing you and being alone was a bit abrupt for me, as you kept your functioning and welcomed others with such excellence and tranquility. I was already too old to carry the two small wheels that was giving support to my bicycle. There are things in life that even if we know, they only exist when we feel them. My bicycle was now at risk of falling, leaning to one side, and it was up to me to keep up the pace so as not to unbalance. I felt a lot of our physical detachment and even jealousy from the other young relationships you were receiving. Luckily, I looked ahead and saw others with whom you had already done the same, and most of them seemed happy to me.

Before I knew, my first supervision of one hundred hours was over, and I was writing the ninety-ninth hour of the second case. I was celebrating like someone celebrating the end of a long marathon and thinking *I am screwed, there goes another small wheel supporting me. What did this mean? Was I now an analyst? Because I conducted two analyses for more than a hundred hours?* You have no idea of the fears I felt and the conviction that it was all too soon and too fast. How much life will still have to show me the anxieties of waiting until an objective and then complaining that it had passed so quickly. At the same time, I didn't want to admit it, it sounded as childish as me asking you to sing a lullaby. I was trying to find that self of mine that was indignant at your orders, and I couldn't find it anymore. I was being congratulated for this step and I had a lot of trouble understanding it. Everything seemed so formal that it made me angry. I wrote to you, how those hours of supervision had been and received what would be the equivalent of a positive thumbs up in *WhatsApp*. In that stormy cloud, between lightning and thunder, my analyst's hand came loose from my bike seat. Even you *Brutus*? After 17 years . . . I know I was complaining, and we had been riding on lukewarm ground lately. But in the middle of the pandemic, we decided to say goodbye, on camera? I don't know what we were thinking, but it was all a bit much for me. An analysis has to be terminable, I know, and spoken like that, it sounds beautiful. The tears from my discharge burned only my face, and for you my dear Institute, it was another necessary step.

Without the two small wheels supporting my bike and now pedaling alone, all I had to do was keep up the momentum so as not to fall. I looked to the sides and saw myself alone. Now the problem was loneliness. I could only perceive unhappy patients, resistance, negative transferences . . . From home to the office, back and forth. I would never admit to missing you at that moment. To conclude this turbulent phase, you formalized what you call graduation. My God, what an irony. When we started, I thought that you would graduate me when I was ready, and now I find out that this is *pro forma*? I don't feel ready and now, what do we do? In fact, there is no such thing as ready or not ready to be an analyst: is this what you wanted me to learn? It is all just steps and more steps, growth and more growth? Adulthood? Is this the cliché repeated endlessly at conferences that we will forever be analysts in training?

There I was, pedaling my bicycle, with no supporting wheels, just the regular two, and no one holding it. Oh, how good it feels to write this, imagining the guilt you must be carrying right now for having done this to me! I admit that despite all the anguish, there was a big part of me that felt proud. It has been a beautiful trajectory up to that point, from the moment we met, to nowadays, graduating after four years of seminars, 200 hours of supervision, reports, and finally, with the termination of my personal analysis. How were we now going to re-establish our communication, our relationship? I had to step back for a while, I learned to enjoy this ride alone, following an uncertain course, but at my own pace. With time, my desperation diminished and to my surprise, when I finally managed to pedal in a more natural way and looked ahead, I saw a fleet of colleagues pedaling on their own as well. They looked at each other, talked to each other, seemed to have turned into a process with less energy expenditure, maybe because they rode in convoy or because their calves were already stronger, I don't know. That's when it hit me that this degree was not the end, but the beginning. I was not yet an analyst. What a relief I felt.

It was then that I remembered our initial arrangement: our relationship would conclude after I showed you what you taught me. You demanded from me a clinical work to be presented, of an analytic process conducted by me and my patient. It was time to formally expose myself, to open up to everyone what these early years of ours had meant. Through this development I could be titled a psychoanalyst, for your and my happiness, I would reach this destination, to join the platoon ahead of me. Suddenly I began to feel your hand pushing my bicycle, making it easier for me to move around, and the peloton ahead grew in size in my field of vision. After forty pages of an analytical report that demonstrated the deepest part of my professional world, I joined the platoon ahead. In this work I exposed as much as possible my relationship with my patient, what I was saying, my theoretical and technical tools, interpretations, and transferences. I tried my best to show you what I was doing between the four walls of my office, wanting us to be proud of my analytical skills, even if they were initial. How I distressed myself thinking that now everyone would know what I look like! When I imagined myself presenting the work to you and everyone else, without exception, I was always naked. Wouldn't there be a way for me to get through it with clothes on? I understood that no, and almost imperceptibly, I realized that your hand was used one last time to fit me into the platoon ahead full of other psychoanalytic colleagues.

It has been difficult for me to put this experience into words. When I reread it, it seems more like the story of a saga. I guess I blame myself a little for not having done it sooner, but we need a relative distance for deeper reflections. We go through an experience, but for me the feelings and thoughts come later. Maybe you feel indignant, because you tried so hard to stay open to hear me while we were together. I am sure we will still meet a lot along the way. Maybe I won't be the one who only drank from your fountain of knowledge and in the future, I could become a colleague at your side, helping to put wheels and hold the bike for others. I don't know, you always made sure to tell me from the beginning that I would start with you, move on, and that this was the way it was supposed to be. Maybe I was not prepared for this emotional roller coaster despite your numerous warnings.

Finally, I want to tell you two things that I also learned during this process. The first refers to the infinite way in which our internal world—conscious/unconscious—interacts with reality. Even though my conscious has to admit by convention that winter is supposed to be cold and two plus two is four, my unconscious doesn't have to. It allows me to feel just like an eternal student for example and it may even consider that I am not a psychoanalyst or, most beautiful of all, allow me to miss something that still exists. When it removes the impoverishing logical thinking of time, I feel free. The second, much more concrete, refers to the psychoanalytic profession. To be linked to an institute and to an association is like waking up every day and eating breakfast so as not to faint, weakened later. Indispensable. There is no psychoanalysis on its own, it is linked with the patient, with colleagues, and with our psyche. It is a profession that works at least in twos, and that in its excellence is accomplished with a much larger portion. Today I consider that while I am analyzing a patient, I am bonding with you, colleagues, analyst, implicit theories, supervisors, and of course my best friend, the patient.

Thank you for giving me a path to a profession.

Greetings,

— Rafael Mondrzak

# 17 A letter to the Finnish Psychoanalytical Society, Helsinki (1964)

*Maria Lival-Juusela*

*The origins of organized psychoanalysis in Finland date back to 1964, when several Finnish analysts who had trained abroad, returned to Finland. They were granted the status of a study group by the Executive Committee of the IPA. Veikko Tähkä was elected chairman with Henrik Carpelan as secretary. The president of the IPA elected Donald W. Winnicott chairman of their sponsoring committee and Pearl King secretary.*

*In 1967 the Finnish Study Group was elevated to the status of a Provisional Society. Two years later it was accepted as a Component Society of the IPA.*

*From 1964 to 1997, the membership of the society grew from 11 to 157. In 2024 there are 177 members and 19 candidates in training. Finland maintains a cooperation with its Nordic neighbors in the Nordic psychoanalytic journal, The Scandinavian Psychoanalytic Review, founded in 1978. The 32nd International Psychoanalytic Congress of the IPA was held in Helsinki in 1981 at Finlandia House. Eero Rechardt was the host and the chairman of the Finnish organizing committee and was elected the vice-president of the IPA 1981–1983. The 5th Scientific Symposium of the European Psychoanalytical Federation was held in 1992 in Helsinki.*

*In Finland, each cohort of candidates follows the same curriculum with training seminars every Friday for four years, and then, more sporadically, for an additional six months. Our cohort, the institute's 32nd, was divided into two groups of eight and nine members. Our training seminars began in August 2018 and ended in January 2023.*

—

Dear Institute,

Thank you for accepting me for training. You made me a candidate, an analyst in training, something I very much wanted to be. Those weeks and months of waiting to hear from you after the application interviews felt like being perched on a threshold, requesting permission to fly. Being accepted or rejected for those "flying lessons" seemed fateful. I don't think I realized all of what it was I wanted. I know I wanted the intellectual and emotional

DOI: 10.4324/9781003465409-17

challenge of training, to deepen my understanding of psychoanalysis from the other side of the couch. I also wanted to belong to a psychoanalytic community, both local and international, to enrich my knowledge of the language and theory and concepts of this pluralistic world and to meet others with similar interests. You seemed to offer all of that. The unconscious reasons I'm still on the path of finding. Why does one want to become an analyst?

"Are you sure? Once you move forward, you can never really go back", my first analyst told me, when as a young student I was deliberating on entering analysis. But I was sure then, and I was sure, scared but sure, twenty years later, applying for training. Dear Institute, I think I wanted more of that same movement my first analysis put me on the path of: to continue swinging on that pendulum between remembering and re-living the past in order to find and enliven the momentum of becoming whoever it was I was on the way of becoming. Of living deliberately, as Thoreau wrote. Twenty years on my wings felt strong enough to allow the dream of bringing others along, while continuing my own analytic journey. "You are moving in the direction of freedom", Toni Morrison once told a graduating class of Barnard, "and the function of freedom is to free somebody else".

Dear Institute, your welcome was warm. In May 2018, you invited us, your 17 new candidates-to-be, to the premises of The Finnish Psychoanalytical Society for introductions and toasts with the training analysts who would teach us. We joked about not knowing which group was the more nervous. The following autumn we began. The two groups studied in adjacent rooms, divided only by glass doors and a small hallway. We could see each other across the hall and sometimes we could hear the other group laugh. We had our lunch break together. I think one of the things you did really well, dear Institute, was impress upon us candidates how important we would become for each other. You encouraged us to make a deliberate effort to that end, to socialize as often as we could. It was a pleasing suggestion—and off we went to theatres and restaurants together. And now, perched on the next threshold—that of graduation and post-graduate planning—we find ourselves sharing a deep sense of the value of continuing to make regular plans together, both professional and social.

Dear Institute, you introduced our cohort to The Finnish Psychoanalytical Society at large during our first year of training. The snow was deep around Lake Tuusula that January and the members and candidates of the society were gathered in a hotel on the frozen lake for our yearly winter-conference. I remember listening to learned and touching papers of fathers and sons and oedipal conflicts, but also to one about you, dear Institute. About what kind of a home that you make for your candidates and members. It was a joined presentation between the two TAs heading our current training program, Ann-Mari Rytöhonka and Henrik Enckell. The presentation described the results of a questionnaire conducted by Ann-Mari Rytöhonka, directed at newly graduated analysts and senior candidates. What had the training seminars given them and how were they faring as analysts? Although the answers were described as diplomatic, as I listened carefully to the presentation, it seemed to carry a tone of warning. While everyone was appreciative of the training seminars, many new analysts also seemed to be feeling alone and vulnerable. Flying solo was surprisingly difficult, especially in the period right after graduating, when the warmth and safety of the training wings came off and societal winds blew cold and unremitting.

In his introduction to the presentation Henrik Enckell quoted a famous line from the Sicilian novel by Giuseppe Tomasi Di Lampedusa, *The Leopard* (1958): "Everything must change for everything to remain the same". In the novel, the ambiguous quote captures both the apparent adaptation to change as well as the deep-seated resistance to it. It is a line uttered by Prince Fabrizio's nephew Tancredi—that is, by a member of the "next generation", trying to navigate his way through momentous societal change. Still the novel's main character is not Tancredi, but his uncle, the prince—ruler of his castle, of his wife, children, servants, mistresses, subjects and dogs. Everyone kisses his ring. But the winds are changing around 19th century Sicily as the republic of Italy is in the process of being born, rocking traditions in their foundations.

Dear Institute, recently, I read *The Leopard*. As I came upon Tancredi's quote again and was reminded of Ann-Mari's and Henrik's presentation at the beginning of my training, I found myself reading the novel almost as a metaphoric story of psychoanalytic institutes themselves, surrounded by the changing societal attitudes toward psychoanalysis.[1] The author Tomasi Di Lampedusa's wife, it must be added, was a psychoanalyst, Alessandra Wolff Stomersee, and Freud's theory, along with the modernist literature of Virginia Woolf and James Joyce, were some of Lampedusa's points of reference in writing. The narrator's tone in the novel is melancholic, tender and wise, unremittingly asking of its characters—again and again—where they stand in the balance between defensive pride and passivity on the one hand and active engagement and open vulnerability on the other, especially in the face of loss. Where they stand in the balance between narcissism and love. How does one remain alive in volatile conditions, especially conditions that push one toward marginality? Applied to psychoanalysis, how does it remain alive as a discipline? How does an institute and the psychoanalytical society that holds it remain a vital home for its members and candidates?

Last summer the editors of this book kindly asked me to contribute a text. These questions of legacy and aliveness were in my mind as I listened to the EPF-congress presentations in Vienna last July and also gave one myself. My paper, given at The Sexual and Gender Diversity Studies workshop, was about mourning the history of the generalized pathologizing of homosexuality within psychoanalysis. Two weeks earlier at Pride Helsinki I had listened as the president of our society, Eija Repo, pronounced a public apology of our society's own history in that regard. Attending the seminar around the apology had been deeply moving, especially after witnessing and partaking in the two-year reflective and cooperative process that preceded it. Listening to an acknowledgement of harm caused and the pronounced wish to accept responsibility for it, to repair and create anew among an audience of many people personally affected, was a moment that felt, quite simply, hopeful. It was an acknowledgement of movement and change over time, of everything *not* having to remain the same. Dear Society, I was so proud of you.

Dear Institute, the sense of hope in a dynamically evolving history within our society felt so deeply sustaining, I believe, because psychoanalytic training is admittedly hard. As candidates we spend our years in training juggling the inevitable varieties of strain: practical, economic, narcissistic, clinical, familial, societal . . . For many candidates just travelling long-distance into Helsinki for the seminars every Friday, by train or plane, is an undertaking. Then, during the first year of training, we practice finding a voice in the group. Spontaneous speaking in a group full of psychoanalytic thinkers isn't always for the faint of heart, as we show ourselves in ways we may not even realize with our utterances—or fear that we do. And then slowly, trust evolves as we realize how much we have in common, as we all begin to tread new professional ground with our first analysands. Until gradually, the ground starts to shake again. The third year, someone warned me, group dynamics are difficult. Everyone's workload is heavy with a multitude of cases and supervisions and the honeymoon of training is over. Projections ricochet across the room.

For my cohort, the end ofthe second and the entirety of the third year of training was also when the pandemic broke out. Suddenly, we lost each other, lost the physical presence, the eye-contact, the invisible nods and bursts of laughter that had helped us recall our own projections. Dear Institute, I know you were as shocked and unprepared as we were in March 2020. I'm grateful that seminars went on so smoothly, even on Zoom, that you scrambled to make that happen, with many TAs teaching for the first time over technology. And yet, of course we felt you dropped us. We were still psychoanalytic chicks, safely tucked in the nest we thought, when the pandemic hit. And even with Zoom, we felt cold and bewildered and much too young to fly alone. Dear Institute, I wish we could have spoken more openly to each other at this point. Mourned more openly together what was happening, all around us in the world, yes, but also, quite specifically, to our training as analysts. I know you must have been bewildered too, yet I wondered at your silence. At the lack of words that hung in the virtual air between all of us, as we met and didn't meet, week after week. The training went on, on Zoom, as we all held our breaths emotionally. Dear Institute, I wish we could have breathed together, right there on Zoom, through that loss, trauma, confusion and sadness and what it did to our training for a time.

In her keynote at the EPF-congress in Vienna last summer the Italian training analyst Paola Marion (2022) spoke of the psychoanalytic legacy we receive and how it must be transformed before it can be possessed. "Together with the Icarus complex, our task is to avoid the Laius complex", said Marion from her perspective of an experienced generation.

If it is not accompanied by the work of mourning, the fall that marks the end of the dream— like the flight of Icarus— tends toward disappointment, results in feelings of rage; pluralism resolves into nihilism and relativism into postmodern nihilism,

she continued. She spoke also of the fundamental human tasks entailed in growing up. The task of each new generation is to make use of, destroy and reinvent the creations of the previous generation. The task of the previous generation is of course to stay alive as we do.

Perhaps it's a question of interpersonal encounters, and navigating those through a history of some rather definite hierarchies? I still wonder at your silences sometimes, dear Institute. How you evaluate us, for instance, or do you? Don't you? You seldom tell me how you see me as an analyst, certainly not systematically. When I ask about this, I'm told it's subjective anyway. I'm sure it is, and that evaluation is difficult. Still, I would have liked to hear more of what you see in my work, the work I show you. I believe it would have been pedagogically deeply useful, and also at times, just plain generous. Your admittedly subjective views matter to me, dear Institute, as I hope mine do to you. I believe that's what mutuality and interpersonal encounters are about, even across hierarchies.

The novel, *The Leopard*, describes the prince's death with an enigmatic metaphor. From behind the mourners around him, suddenly a young woman in a brown travelling dress makes her way to his deathbed, to raise the veil of her straw hat and meet the prince's gaze, as all sound around him subsides. It's a scene that can be understood in many ways— perhaps this woman is a mirage, a phantasy, of a dying man, reaching for a last encounter after a lifetime of forfeited mutuality. But what I took from it was this: Dear Institute, I think staying alive takes two. I think the movement from death to rebirth *requires* that asymmetry and chafing between youth and experience. Perhaps it carries in itself an acknowledgment of temporality, of both undeniable demise and the promise of renewal. I think it needs a lifted veil; a gaze that meets and challenges the gaze of the other, even, maybe especially, in the face of mortality and painful transformation. I agree that staying alive needs mourning, but I also think it needs a multitude of travelling companions, because, quite simply, that's what makes it *fun*. Perhaps one does become an analyst to continue to search for answers about oneself, but I also don't think one becomes an analyst unless one deeply enjoys engaging with other people. The pandemic certainly brought that lesson home. It shook us in our foundations by showing us how much we truly need each other to do this job well, how much becoming and working as an analyst is dependent on fellowship. Companionship. Not on kissing the static ring of hierarchical history, but on debating it, transforming it and carrying it forward in a myriad of ways together.

Now more than ever, I think societies need their members and candidates engaged, just as we need societies and institutes that don't shrink from what those generational and fraternal bonds, truly, madly, deeply, ask of us. Perhaps we create a home for each other by surrendering, again and again, to the pluralistic dialectics we all represent by debating, killing off, repairing, working through, creating anew. Not just on and behind the couch, but among ourselves. For that, I think we have to put on our travelling dresses and *show up*, unafraid to challenge our history, each other and ourselves.

And then, dear Institute, we fly.

— Maria Lival-Juusela

## Note

1 Warm thanks to fellow candidate, Giuseppe Caruso, training at the British Psychoanalytical Society for discussions on this topic and for explaining the novel's significance from a Sicilian point of view. And especially for debating with me and showing me how the parallel I draw between the novel and psychoanalytic institutes both works and doesn't work. *Il Gattopardo* is a Sicilian novel, that describes how the arrogance and decadent choices of the Sicilian aristocracy tragically contribute to the miseries and poverty of the majority of Sicilians, the fateful consequences of which persist to this day. This pessimistic view is certainly not the parallel I'm after. For the sake of my argument here, I am making use of the novel's universal and psychological themes: the sense in which "we are all Sicilians", i.e. resistant to change and at risk of being corrupted or seduced by power and charisma within hierarchies.

# 18 A letter to the Association Psychanalytique de France, Paris (1964)

## Samuel Lannadère

*Basic requirements for graduating from the APF (Association Psychanalytique de France):*

- *Two control cases*
- *One paper on a third case, conducted without control, which will be presented by the candidate to the training commission*
- *Being able to account for institutional participation, specifically study-groups throughout your whole candidacy*

*In France the history of psychoanalytical associations is one of conflicts. The APF is the result of two successive divisions from the first association that existed in the country. These divisions have carved the structure of the training in the APF. The first one was one for autonomy from what was considered as the hierarchal teaching of the primary association. Leaving the IPA-affiliated association, the dissidents consequently were ousted from the IPA. This division was conducted by Daniel Lagache and Jacques Lacan. The second one was initiated for two reasons. Taking distance from Lacan and his grasp on the newly formed association was thought necessary, the main reason, however, was to reenter the IPA. This second division was the birth of the APF.*

*This beginning is at the heart of the complex relationship between teaching and training at the APF.*

*We are reminded there that psychoanalysis cannot be book-taught, or even taught for that matter. In this regard, the Institute offers few workgroups in its own name, in fear that we candidates might think them as compulsory or maybe that we would consider this teaching as satisfying minimum technical knowledge.*

*Every year, the institute organizes a gathering of the candidates to talk specifically about teachings at the APF. For the past three years, it has come down on the one hand to the appreciation of the performativity of any proposition coming down from the institute and on the other hand to question furthermore what could be considered as a handing down of psychoanalysis itself, aside from the personal analysis. In one of the gathering I mentioned, a candidate accurately said that he thought an analytical teaching wasn't about learning something, it is about having one's relationship to knowledge altered.*

DOI: 10.4324/9781003465409-18

*The APF Institute, doesn't fall short. It encourages candidates—even newly accepted ones—and members to form study-groups to keep on questioning the analytical epistemology and its connection to the cure, the furthest away possible from any type of control on knowledge.*

—

Dear institute,

As I planned to write something on what I might expect from you—and thought this letter an easy one—I couldn't begin, being stopped each time by the fact that I was to address you as "dear". I found starting this letter calling a psychoanalytical institute "dear" rather puzzling—politeness, manners, and customs notwithstanding.

The relationship I entertain with you—and I think any candidate does—is all but an unequivocal one. It is highly ambivalent. This ambivalence however should not be discarded as the mere unavoidable and necessary caution that comes with any application to an institution because therein lies the complexity of my relationship to psychoanalysis and its handing down itself.

I think it is deeply linked to the reasons I applied.

As a clinical psychologist I was, before my candidacy, already enabled to take into my care patients anyway I thought fit. The five years I spent in university allowed me to study the theory and being in a psychoanalytically oriented university, the theory I studied was Freud's and his many disciples. I had undergone controls for several therapies and could have been supervised for an analysis, should I have chosen to lie down a patient. Conferences and study-groups are not hard to come by in Paris. So why candidate?

For sure, I needed a sense of affiliation that I thought only you could offer.

You specifically question the connection between theory and practice. It has been very important for me to learn to stand clear from any type of grip on patients—even ones coming from knowledge. Distinguish epistemology as hard knowledge from theory as representation is a difficulty you help me address.

But, dear institute, can someone be an analyst without knowing any theory?

In radical terms of transference interpretation, I would think someone—who has undergone an analysis himself—can. That's why I think the primary condition to apply to an psychoanalytical institute is a nonnegotiable one: the experience that the interpretation of transference is one of deep transformation. This is also how I understand the frame of the training at any API affiliated association: the control by a member of at least two cures. In my opinion, the only passing on of psychoanalysis itself is the experience of the analytical cure.

The issue of knowledge, and thus of being taught by an institute, revolves, I would say, around two perspectives: a clinical and an epistemological one.

It is certain that some clinical experience is absolutely needed in order to be an analyst. One should be able to recognize nosographical signs that prevent us to lay down a patient, or to address him to a colleague should the patient need medication or hospitalization. If this clinical knowledge is not yours to teach, it is your responsibility to make sure that candidates have the necessary clinical background.

If knowing is not ground for analytical entitlement, I think being able to talk about our patients, to share experience is at the heart of our practice—which is a lonely one.

Between the analyst and the patient, theory acts as a third party. I think having colleagues to argue with, to confront my own understanding of the Freudian's theory is necessary. Metapsychology, in Freud's words, is our mythology, and our very own transference on theory is always to be questioned, for it is always a risk that we forget that the analytical theory is merely a representation of the analytical process and not the process in itself.

This is what you can provide: offering candidates the means to interpret our transference on theory. This is of importance because the way we understand the theory has a direct impact on the way we practice. The theory we continue to elaborate as candidates, and I would reckon as members as well, its endeavor to articulate something on human beings as subjects of their own madness is always connected to the experience of the unconscious, and thus to sexuality. The scandal of psychoanalysis will never be a thing of the past. Dear Institute, you have the difficult task to both try to protect us from its possible individual repercussions and to prevent its dilution.

One more office you have for me is to keep alive some of the questions I addressed to psychoanalysis itself as I began my own cure. Bearer of the complexity of my relationship to the method and its efficiency, you are, in my mind, the legitimate institution to consider the doubts, the loneliness and the despair that sometimes come with the impossible job of being an analyst. All of these should not aggrieve patients and you are needed there as a third party, shielding them from too much hatred, or too much love.

The many functions I dare say you uphold are the very reasons one should hear the two meanings of the word "dear" when referred to you: both appreciated and onerous.

The narcissistic satisfactions of being accepted in the training are pretty clear: I found myself grateful and pleased to become a candidate. The Institute offers possibilities of camaraderie and learning, the association a sense of belonging. Those are easily cherished.

On the other hand, many aspects of the candidacy appear at times unnerving: the weight of the institution itself, its often vertical-functioning, the rivalry between members or the expectations you may legitimately—or not—have, as well as the disillusions that necessarily followed the somewhat idealized version I had before I applied or even the fear of a loss of originality or independence. All of which contribute to consider you as costly.

You are indeed very dear.

— Samuel Lannadère

# 19 A letter to the Oregon Psychoanalytic Center, Portland, United States of America (1965)

*Cynthia (Cindi) Palman*

*The Oregon Psychoanalytic Center (OPC) has had a tradition of excellence since its earliest origins as the Oregon Study Group, which began in 1965; it was accepted by the American Psychoanalytic Association (APsaA) as a study group in 1981 and as a society in 1994. In 1995 Oregon Psychoanalytic Institute (OPI) was established as a new training facility under the auspices of APsaA and the sponsorship of the San Francisco Psychoanalytic Institute. In 2005 the Oregon Psychoanalytic Institute was granted status as a provisional institute, and in 2010 it became a freestanding APsaA institute. Its collaboration with San Francisco continues in the areas of teaching and consultation. In July 2003, the Oregon Psychoanalytic Society and Institute merged with Oregon Psychoanalytic Foundation to form the Oregon Psychoanalytic Center, providing a new model for expanding psychoanalytic ideas and psychotherapy in the community.*

*The graduation requirements for Oregon Psychoanalytic are as follows:*

*(i) Three cases, two for over two years and one for one year.*
*(ii) 1,200 hours of sessions with patients.*
*(iii) Weekly supervision for all three cases.*
*(iv) Three final case reports of each analysis and the blessing of the progression committee determining you are ready.*

—

Dear Institute,

Sitting in the flux between candidate and graduate analyst I am aware of the prayer in me "not to get lost." No longer do I have our didactic classes to anchor my place here. My class is spreading out like a drop of ink expanding in water. My classmates wonder about their future place in this family—imagine moving on in their search for a psychic home. I call us a family because that is what I, and many others, are looking for when we make our way to becoming a candidate, a family that understands a "something" we have felt all our lives that has always made us feel a little bit different; the need to be

DOI: 10.4324/9781003465409-19

with others in an emotional and psychological intimacy. We arrive at your doorstep looking for others who feel compelled to understand ourselves, our families and the drama of human existence.

So, what I wish to speak to you about is the survival of this family, our institute, and the field beyond, because I am very grateful that you are here and you gave me the opportunity to learn about becoming an analyst. Dear institute—we all know families are full of tensions but at their best they provide a place of security through acceptance; acceptance of the individual, of our differences, of conflicts and tensions, of the need to grow and spread one's wings, and the passing of the torch from one generation to the next. They need to survive the discovery of new ideas each generation must make, while holding on to the traditions and history that provide the bedrock for this growth. Our institutes need to be a good enough container to hold all these fiery tensions and allow us to come together in functioning working groups.

Dear institute, I believe one problem is the privileging of the dyad in our training and our profession even though we all live in groups, e.g., family of origin, new family, professional groups etc. I think this privileging of the dyad limits us clinically and leaves our institutes and our professional associations vulnerable to strife and division. The intimacy and secrecy of our dyads draw us in, perhaps recalling the early infant-mother bond. We feel protected from the chaos of the outside world and take comfort in the safety of the couple. Preserving this safety is important for the training analysis and supervisions, but I think there is an over privileging of the dyads in psychoanalysis at the expense of appreciating the function of the groups that are present in analytic training and within our analytic community. We value the couples of the analyst/analysand, and supervisor/supervisee more than we do candidate cohorts, faculty groups or analytic community. Protecting these dyads also protects us from the anxiety of separation and the array of feelings that come with it. Of course, our work requires the health of these dyads, but forgetting about the group leaves our analytic communities vulnerable. Information about the larger group may be held within the individual pairings, but not looked at collectively. Tensions and conflict are left to grow. I believe COVID exposed this vulnerability as it did with so many other cracks in our society. Engaging in analytic work can be taxing. We all depend on the support and superego of the group to engage in this workday after day. When our community can provide these functions, we can all be more resilient and creative.

Dear institute, my cohort was not one of the lucky classes that formed a bond that strengthened and expanded the learning experience. Our identity as a group was shaky prior to COVID, unable to work with the expected dynamics that occur when you launch eight successful professionals back to childhood. When we would bring up our class tension with supervisors or peers, you dismissed it as endemic to candidate classes. Then COVID descended and our teachers, analysts, and supervisors seemed to move overnight to Zoom, looking for personal safety and the survival of the work. Our Institute members had very little experience teaching and working online.

Although community meetings were offered monthly, I don't think anyone realized what effect this was having on my class. Certainly, our supervisors and analysts heard some of our distress in their dyadic meetings, but there wasn't a collective attention where our story could be put together. The stress and separation of the pandemic seemed to shatter what connection my class had and with this destroyed our ability to learn together; to be generous and giving of our feeling-thoughts. I believe group generativity is an essential component of learning to think analytically. I wish you had done more to create an atmosphere where we were free enough to connect experientially with the concepts we were studying. We needed to be able to play with new ideas, in much the same way we're asking our patients to play with new ideas. Your silence made us retreat further inward.

The necessity of a functioning group and, I believe, in person learning, for analytic education was demonstrated during our final year of didactic classes. We returned to in person classes because you agreed with us on the importance of in the in person learning experience. In addition, you heard our distress and agreed to provide us with a consultant to work on our group process. Through this work our ability to creatively and authentically engage with each other came to light. We learned more from each other than in the previous three years, not just in the group process but in all of our classes. We found out how as individuals and as a group we could tolerate anger, envy, and disagreement. This made it possible to bring more of ourselves into the room and into the creative engagement with each other. The deadness of our Zoom room was replaced with an alive and lively classroom.

I end this letter with thanks and a challenge. I wish to express my gratitude for the hundreds of hours you have contributed to our education and for returning to "live" classes before the rest of the country. I would like to encourage you to rethink the privileging of the dyad and recognize the necessity of attending to the perhaps more difficult, and certainly less private, realm of the group as essential to psychoanalytic learning and a vibrant community. Dear institute—recognize that the "didactic" leg of our tripartite model is also the group experiential learning. That the functioning group environment helps us to both think and feel the ideas we are learning beyond the intellectual level. Prepare new candidate classes in group work and invite them into our community from the beginning. Commit our faculty to engaging in this experiment. Support them with trainings. Attend to group dynamics in all of our committees and classrooms, not as the primary focus, but to function as an internal backbone to make the work in committee and classroom possible. Although some education on groups is involved, I think this is more a change in attitude and attention, then the creation of a new training model. While we are comprised of wonderful, giving, and caring individuals, at times we have difficulties joining together as a functional working group, and we become suspicious, divided, and more vulnerable to fears about our survival. Giving us a "group" backbone will allow us to recover quickly when the basic assumptions begin to dominate, as happens in all groups. And because

I believe we need to be in the same room and share the same air to work together, I ask that you don't give up on our "in person" community. I know you are experiencing the struggles that many small institutes face in USA. I believe by embracing the importance of in person learning as an essential element of psychoanalytic education, we can not only survive, but thrive and excel in our programming. We can continue to be proud of what Oregon Psychoanalytic Institute has to offer. Let's be that welcoming and accepting family that is able to promote the ongoing study and development of this very living journey we call psychoanalysis.

— Cynthia (Cindi) Palman

# 20 A letter to Institut für Psychoanalyse und Psychotherapie Freiburg, Germany (1965)

*Sebastian Thrul*

*The Institut für Psychoanalyse und Psychotherapie Freiburg (IPPF) developed out of a working group of the German Psychoanalytical Society (DPG) in the 1960s. The institute has always been active, creative and well connected to many mental health institutions in the area. One very important and productive feature of the institute is the jointly training of analysts working with adults and analysts working with children and adolescents. Both respective vantage points greatly enrich clinical and theoretical discussions.*

*Unfortunately, like many psychoanalytic and psychotherapeutic institutions, the institute has a regrettable history of authoritarian leadership and abuse of power that explicitly or implicitly has to be worked through by each subsequent generation of psychoanalysts in training. Although I did not consciously set out to do so in the following letter to the institute, I can see in hindsight how I am implicitly addressing the institute's history in it.*

*My institute follows the requirements of the German Psychoanalytic Society (DPG):*

- *I have to be in my own training analysis for the duration of training with a frequency of at least three sessions per week in the classical (couch) setting.*
- *I have to do two supervised control analyses in the classical (couch) setting with a frequency of at least three sessions per week, running for at least 250 sessions each.*
- *I also have to do four additional "modified" supervised control treatments with a lower frequency and in a non-classical setting (sitting up).*
- *I have to attend theoretical and clinical seminars throughout training.*

—

Dear Institute,

When I first started out in psychoanalytic training, one of your senior analysts uttered a shocking and provocative statement in a theoretical seminar:

DOI: 10.4324/9781003465409-20

"A psychoanalyst never apologizes!" I was taken aback. Granted, it was a tongue-in-cheek statement, presented as a hand-me-down from a previous generation. Nevertheless, it came up in a discussion about a clinical situation in which an analyst was late for a session. Consciously, and outwardly, I was dismayed! What derisive grandiosity the statement seemed to transpire! Such arrogance shall not stand, I thought, and so I argued and argued against it. I cannot remember much of the actual discussion, only my internal process that followed from it—let me tell you about it.

I had started my psychoanalytic training shortly after I had started my psychiatric training. So I had started out seeing patients in various psychiatric settings, not really being prepared for the intensity of the contacts I was confronted with. In those early clinical days, I could observe myself in private moments drinking from the exact well that I had decried as poisoned: "An analyst never apologizes!" In the heat of a number of clinical encounters, when I was confronted with intense hatred from patients and bitter accusations were levelled against me, the grandiosity of the statement provided a sense of comfort. No matter how small and inept I felt, no matter how hard the reproaches hit me—wasn't I also en route to becoming an analyst, that supreme being, that was somehow above the petty day-to-day and perfectly equipped to always take the high ground?

Does an analyst never apologize, because he is always right? Just as a physician never apologizes, because he is always right? I wondered. This sentiment seemed to tally with my socialization as a medical doctor who is supposed to know best, to not make mistakes. Most of us candidates come with a similar training background. In medicine, just as in psychology, you learn how to be certain about matters, either from a perspective of algorithm and diagnoses, or from a perspective of statistics and data. So, dear senior analysts, you must keep in mind that we come to psychoanalysis with the baggage of a sense that we need to be right. And I must tell you, you have given me more than enough reasons to believe that you also at times share this belief.

I will never forget a public clinical discussion at one of the first psychoanalytic conferences I attended. One of you had prepared case notes on a very difficult treatment that left him uncertain, and overwhelmed. To this day, it has been a rare occurrence in my training that one of you should make themselves publicly vulnerable like that, so I was full of awe. The presentation started out well enough, as the presenting analyst had devised a format that befitted his need for a facilitating environment: He would present some notes for a few minutes, and then the audience would respond with associations to the material. In the blink of an eye, however, the discussion with the whole audience deteriorated to a back-and-forth between the presenting analyst and a handful of seemingly masterful and skillful clinicians and dignitaries in the first row, who all seemed to know each other by name and who told everybody else how "it" is done.

Well, I exaggerate. And to be sure, there is more than enough oedipal material here on my part to justify dismissing this experience right off the bat. Do give this some thought though, dear senior analysts: How often do you succumb to the temptation of public grandiosity and certainty? We all drink from that well, from time to time. Best to analyze it, wouldn't you agree? Don't we share the belief that every attempt at mastery is thwarted by the unconscious, and that we would do well to accept our castration? After all, this acknowledgement opens up new routes for solidarity, new vistas for cooperative discovery.

To be sure, there were other instances, mostly in more intimate settings, where some of you were indeed willing to humbly acknowledge the workings of the unconscious and try to use them to deepen clinical exploration. When I had just started an analytic treatment in the classical setting, I brought that zeal for mastery to supervision. I was able to secure supervision with one of you whose clinical acumen, knowledge and experience I admired greatly. I wrote transcript after transcript of the first sessions with the analysand. I worked so hard. I tried to impress the supervisor, and to facilitate the deepest understanding possible. He tried to slow me down a bit, to tell me that I did not have to work quite so hard, that understanding would develop over time. There was, however, some mixed messaging—or at least, mixed message receiving—going on. I felt criticized quite a lot, whenever I was told that I did not see something or that I focused too much on one aspect—the transference, the affect, my reverie—of the clinical encounter to the omission of other aspects. So while the attempts at slowing me down were going on, at the same time I felt called to master the clinical situation better, which lead to more overzealous acceleration on my part. This went on for quite a while, until the supervisor managed to reach me not by more theoretical explanations or demands, but, oddly enough, by a slip. While talking about the analysand in supervision, the supervisor said "I", instead of "he", the analysand. There was a perplexed moment of silence, followed by roaring and joyous laughter by the supervisor, followed again by relieved chuckling on my part. In retrospect, I felt like this revered supervisor had given me a great gift by allowing himself to slip. I don't remember the theoretical explanation that developed from this scene. I do, however, remember the feeling of relief and gratitude that followed from the shared experience, acknowledgement and appreciation of the workings of the unconscious signified by the slip that brought out an unconscious identification of the supervisor with the analysand.

It is in moments like these in which I appreciate you greatly, dear senior analysts—less for the "training" you give me, but for the formative experience you provide me with.

I won't let you off the hook that easily though. Not just yet.

Acknowledging and celebrating a slip, a "mistake" that did not harm anyone, and that happened in an intimate setting, is not really a tall order. But you have to start somewhere, I guess.

Let me tell you some more about my clinical development. After having worked for years and years in psychiatric settings, I was finally about to become a psychiatric "senior physician"—although, in the psychoanalytic world, I was still a toddler. Be that as it may, the psychiatric institution I work for asked whether I would be willing to take on the responsibility of creating and running a clinic for gender dysphoric and trans patients, together with one experienced analyst who had already worked in this area for a long time. Although I was flattered by the offer, I was also terrified. I could not imagine any other field of public discourse that was equally riddled with controversy. After I had ambivalently accepted the challenge, my first impulse was an attempt at—yes, you guessed it—mastery. Before even my first clinical encounter with a trans person, I thought I should read and read and read everything I could about the subject. I felt the weight of the mistakes that you and those that came before you have made in excluding and preemptively pathologizing gender variant people. I spend countless hours to devise elaborate ways of addressing my prospective patients properly. I thought a lot about how it might be possible to keep them out of harm's way as soon as they set foot in the psychiatric institution, to minimize the risk for misgendering or other uncomfortable confrontations. I invested all that energy because I felt it pertinent to do right by people who have been harmed by our discourses and actions for generations. I felt remorseful. But most of all, I think, I wanted to protect myself. I'll come back to that.

What really helped when I was confronted with the daunting task of setting up the clinic was the fact that I was still in my own analysis. The impulse to read all that I could was easily analyzed as a defense against the anxiety provoked by any ordinary psychoanalytic encounter combined with the fact that it was to be, at the same time, an encounter within an at times acrimonious public discourse. So I left the books and the papers aside, for now, and braced for the impact of the clinical situation. And let me tell you, it wasn't that bad. I realized that I was sufficiently equipped through my psychoanalytic training, through my own analysis and supervision, with your help, to work with trans people. The surrounding controversies pushed into the consulting room as well, though, and I found myself in some very difficult situations where, for example, I was severely admonished by patients for even asking questions about their life in general, when all they wanted was a letter that they were indeed trans and could go for somatic transitional procedures. In my work with some of these people, my feeling of remorse made way for something different, that in retrospect I could probably describe as grandiosity. I did start to read some authors who seemed to provide a very clear image of trans people as severely disturbed individuals. Their transness, according to some authors, was simply a defense against underlying, more complex issues. In my most beleaguered moments, these grandiose statements that oftentimes did not take into account the clinicians' countertransference, or indeed, their own transference, seemed to ease my anxieties—I wasn't doing anything wrong; the patients were just very disturbed.

So, remorse and grandiosity made strange bedfellows. How could I understand the simultaneous impulses to bow and grovel *and* to grandiosely distance myself from the objects I was confronted with? I did not understand, for quite a while.

Something odd happened in my own analysis, not that long ago, and while I was still struggling with my questions about my reactions to trans people.

My analyst forgot about me. It sounds awful when I put it like that, so let me explain. I had asked to re-arrange the time for some of my sessions, as my schedule had become crowded due to my growing clinical responsibilities. My analyst graciously accommodated me. And then it happened: She did not show up on time for one of our sessions, and I had to ring her to remind her of the newly arranged time. I was furious! The first thing she did when she arrived at the scene was apologize—which only intensified my rage! Remember, analysts don't apologize, and how dare she dampen my justified anger! We had been working for years by then, and I felt comfortable enough to rave and rage for a while. Then I told her that she had better #@%$! deal with what had led to her forgetting me, and that was that. Until it happened again. And again. Over the course of a few months. I had no idea what to make of it, and I grew tired of getting angry. I was also a bit concerned. Was she getting old?

And then something even more disorienting happened: One day, she ended a session before it was time. I knew it right when I got up from the couch. Although I do not have a watch on me in the consulting room, I found that I have developed a very keen sense of time during the analytic hour, and I can usually tell pretty accurately when it is time to stop. It wasn't time to stop. She ended the session anyway. Stunned, I got out of the room, opened the front door and got out of the building. Checked my watch. I was right! She had kicked me out prematurely! What the @#%$!? I thought only Lacanians did that? I was standing there, unsure what to do.

Moments later, the door of her building opened once more and out she came. "I have ended the session too early!"—"Yeah, well . . ."—"*Scheisse!*", she exclaimed forcefully. Again, I was stunned. I had never experienced her outside of her building, let alone using strong language. It was oddly comforting, seeing her disoriented, taken out of her comfortable chair, and very obviously feeling bad about what had happened. She never apologized, but I could see that she was very sorry for having cut my session short. This was not about her, not about her wish to be forgiven, she was just genuinely sorry she had done something bad to me—it was about me. I don't doubt that she analyzed for herself what had happened. I, however, needed no explanations and apologies. I was content to see her struggle and deal with her guilt herself.

And that, dear senior analysts, is the difference between remorse and guilt, at least to my mind. I could make sense of this difference after attending a theoretical discussion, in which one of you raised the issue of differentiating between remorse and guilt. Remorse, just like grandiosity, seems to be about protecting a fragile self. The wish to be forgiven stabilizes the self when guilt is felt to be unbearable. Guilt, on the other hand, is profoundly about the object. In a mature position of guilt, one doesn't shirk away from questions of how exactly one has damaged it and how to make reparations.

How exactly did this situation help me with my trans patients? Well, it didn't—at least not in any concrete sense. It was an experience that combined with a theoretical elaboration and helped me to make sense of something I had preconsciously grasped at before. As I said above, my psychoanalytic training feels more like a series of formative events than a clear guidebook. We don't trade in manuals and clear-cut interventions. The scene with my analyst, just like many other scenes I experienced with you, opened up space in me. They made me understand that I neither needed to be apologetic about being a psychoanalyst who is interested in the whole person, nor did I need to ride off on a high horse and analyze from afar. I needed to be present for the struggle of initiating and facilitating processes of deeper exploration that is necessarily embedded in a dependable relationship.

So, I think that in the best moments, analytic training has helped me to develop internal space—most of all, for my own struggles with myself, that get actualized to a certain degree in each and every clinical encounter. The development and continual maintenance of this internal space keeps me from actively harming my patients by giving up the analytic position, either by being too close and remorseful, or too detached and grandiose.

"A psychoanalyst never apologizes!" When at first, I was torn between public rejection of this statement, and a private intoxication by its grandiosity, I am now still of two minds, but also somehow less interested in it. What I learned from the experiences described above was that a sense of guilt is not necessarily signified by an apology. What might be most needed from analysts in instances where they should feel guilty, is analyzing. The best aspects of training enable me to bear guilt, to use it productively to understand my reactions to our patients better and to differentiate between my own transference and countertransference. You helped me understand that we don't get the sweet relief of an apology, of asking for forgiveness. We self-analyze, and then we analyze the patient. To that end, we must forgo the desire to masochistically bow and grovel, or to sadistically put all our problems on the patient.

I am so grateful that some of you, dear senior analysts, have allowed me glimpses of your own struggles with grandiosity, remorse and guilt. In your best moments, you showed me how to bear the guilt of one's own fuck-ups and destructivity graciously and how to use both productively. I have personally and professionally profited greatly from the moments when you did not deny your failures, and let me attack you for them, and stayed alive, and did not plot revenge, but kept wondering, and thinking, and analyzing.

It is a shame that not more of you bring your capacities to the public sphere. We are in desperate need of role models who show us how to deal with destruction of other people and the environment neither with grandiosity, nor with shallow remorse, but with actual guilt and concern for the object. But maybe that is for our generation to carry back to the public.

— Sebastian Thrul

# 21 A letter to the Mexican Association for the Practice, Research and Teaching of Psychoanalysis, Mexico City (1965)

*Susana Maldonado Ponce*

*To understand the history of the Mexican Association for the Practice, Research and Teaching of Psychoanalysis (AMPIEP), it is necessary to take into account that, in Mexico, psychologists, anthropologists and educators were excluded and did not have the possibility of studying psychoanalysis.*

*In 1957, when APM (Mexican Psychoanalytic Association) was founded, three psychologists, a criminologist and social worker and a doctor were invited to collaborate with them. Three years later, the collaboration of the four non-physicians was suspended, but they were still interested in training as psychoanalysts. In 1964, a colleague of theirs, Frida Rosenberg, was also looking for serious training and, perhaps, to open a path for psychologists.*

*After several meetings that began in September 1964, the Mexican Association of Psychotherapy was constituted on April 27, 1965. The surname Psychoanalytic was forbidden by APM, as well as the use of the divan. Using the words psychoanalytic psychotherapy was considered the ultimate daring. Changing the name to Mexican Association of Psychoanalytic Psychotherapy (AMPP), was not carried out until April 25, 1973, that is, eight years later.*

*Training in Psychoanalysis began with the group of women founders, who were: Raquel Berman, Felisa Poveda, Vidalina Ramos, Frida Rosenberg, Beatriz Rosas and Dolores M. de Sandoval.*

*Thus, AMP was the first institution to offer training in psychoanalysis for non-medical professionals, since the first Psychoanalytic Circle, which claims to be the first to have offered this type of studies, was formed in August 1969, including the Emaus Psychoanalytic Center, which was also important in the development of non-medical psychoanalysis in Mexico, was founded on April 25, 1966.*

*The Sigmund Freud Institute is a commission of the Board of Directors of the Association where training in psychoanalysis began.*

*After this, the five founders, already graduated, immediately constituted a new Technical Council and took charge of the organization and the different functions. In 1973, they legally changed the name of the Mexican Association of Psychotherapy to the Mexican Association of Psychoanalytic Psychotherapy (AMPP).*

DOI: 10.4324/9781003465409-21

In 1983, a two-year course in Psychodynamics was instituted, which later became the master's degree in Psychoanalytic Research.

In 1987, AMPP joined the North American Council for Psychoanalytic Psychotherapists of New York.

Since 1988, Raquel Berman spearheaded efforts to join the International Psychoanalytic Association (IPA), which was achieved by July 2009 and made official in January 2010.

AMPP's application was denied in 2005 because the name of the Association did not make it clear that it was an eminently psychoanalytic Institution, as it had psychotherapy in its name. The name had to be changed again and as of May 2006 we are the Mexican Association for the Practice, Research and Teaching of Psychoanalysis (AMPIEP). The decision to change the name was approved in the Assembly of February 15, 2006.

—

Dear Institute,

Wow, where to start . . . I'm sitting here and I begin to experience a whirlwind of emotions and ideas. The first word that comes to my mind when I think of AMPIEP *(Mexican Association for the Practice, Research and Teaching of Psychoanalysis)* is **gratitude.** During the four years of training, I met the most wonderful teachers/analysts, which I can describe as empathic, human and kind. I never felt alone even though the path became rough sometimes. What I like the most about my Institute (which was one of the reasons why I chose to study there) is that the attention is really personalized, the groups are small (my group started with six people, ended the seminars four of us) and we are treated as persons, not just as one more student. I remember the three interviews I had before entering the training; I was so nervous! It was hard, I remember leaving one interview thinking "what has just happened?!", I left other interview really angry and went straight to my analysis to figure out what was starting to move inside of me. I realized I still had a long, long way to go in my personal analysis.

So, the journey began with six people. After one semester, one candidate couldn't continue and left the training, halfway of the training another candidate had personal difficulties and also left the training, so four women were together in this path. Four women at different points in their lives: a woman with two teenage children, another one married, another one who started the training pregnant and finished it with her baby in her arms and me, the youngest one, which created a lot of insecurity in me since I was constantly asking myself if I could handle everything that comes with becoming a psychoanalyst. I felt that I lacked a lot of life experience, maturity . . . I was scared. However, the four of us had a life project in common, we were united by our passion for psychoanalysis and we also created very deep and genuine bonds. Thanks to this support I can say that I managed to get through the nights of anguish, the times of regression, the moments of anger and disappointment. That's when I understood the importance of the group. There were long nights where we encouraged each other to continue with the readings, we shared doubts, uncertainty but also emotion, illusion and affection.

After some time at the institute, I realized there were many aspects I didn't know existed, for example politics. I didn't know anything about political issues or how institutes worked, so I started hearing that weekly there were board meetings and that's where all the projections and persecution started. My fantasies were *"are they talking about us? what are they saying? why is everything so secret and why can't they share with us what they talk in those meetings?"* Yes, my super ego was starting to personalize in this *"strange, and ethereal mass"* called *"the board of directors".* Among our group we even laughed about this and made jokes like imagining them as witches with their cauldron deciding our future as analysts (of course this was a way to ease our persecution).

The moment of truth came at the end of each semester, where we received group feedback by each of our teachers, and then we were called personally to talk with them about our performance during that semester. Then, after some weeks, we received a letter that gathered a qualitative description of all the teachers we had during the semester. Yes, almost all the times I felt really angry with something they described about me. Sometimes I even felt like they didn't know me at all or that they didn't notice my efforts, but with time and hard work in personal analysis I could understand what they were trying to tell me. As the institute worked many times as a projection target, I was really mad about having to wait maybe one or two months for the letter. In my regression I started acting like a child making a tantrum and I remember saying to my analyst something like *"It's not fair! Just because you have the power you can't play with our time! If we have to submit a paper for your class it must be on time, so why don't you do the same! It's disrespectful!"* What I didn't see at that time was the enormous work all the analysts do at my institute. As I just mentioned, maybe one of the most hard parts of being in the training is the enormous regression that is experimented, that's why for me having my personal analysis, supervisions, seminars and my group of peers was the key to endure this long and hard journey. Several times I remember crying at night, asking myself if all this hard work was really worth it. The answer is **YES**.

When I remember my seminars, all I can do is smile. I liked so much the dynamic where we discussed the lectures we read and we could feel free to ask questions, even to share personal examples and everyone was respectful. Of course, not all seminars were great, I didn't like some classes, but nothing can be perfect. The class that I liked the most was group supervision, where each semester one candidate presented a patient and transcribed sessions, it was really an amazing experience. We had the opportunity to have online seminars before the pandemic with analysts from other parts of the world so that was awesome.

After two years of training, we started hearing about IPSO and OCAL so I became IPSO representative and a whole new adventure began at that moment. I started creating bonds with other candidates and assisting to congresses, that changed my whole training experience. I was angry that my Institute didn't tell us about this organizations but for my surprise they didn't know the importance of this. As my colleagues and me started transmitting them what this was about, my Institute fully supported and encouraged the new generations to become members.

Something that marked my training was that in 2017 a big earthquake hit Mexico City, many buildings collapsed, it was chaotic. Mental health was needed because of the enormous losses people had. As a young and energetic woman, I started acting in a maniac way trying to "help" but in the wrong way, I had to stop and analyze what was happening to me, because I felt really angry at my institute when they said to me *"stop, we have to wait, analyze the situation and protect ourselves in order to help in the best moment and manner".* I remember my confusion and disappointment; I couldn't understand why they were so "passive". After some months I realized they were being careful and they were planning a strategy to help. They planned support groups for people who needed to talk about what happened, they gave us a crisis intervention course to have tools to help in an analytical way but in a different way. So, each candidate was in a group with a senior analyst. After each session, candidate and analyst talked about what happened in the group and tried to process the emotions. It was not easy because we were in a parallel situation, we were also affected by the earthquake. This was a breaking point where the sense of helping the community took importance to me. I knew my institute had a long history prioritizing the help in the community mostly helping women suffering from gender violence, they even won the IPA in the Community Award about Violence in 2019 with their work entitled *"Normalized gender violence introjected in Mexican female identity,"* but this time it really made an impact on me.

Talking about the official supervisions, I really liked both experiences, but it was so exhausting having to make the transcript of the sessions! I thought *"why do they want to torture us? Why can't they see that we have many lectures to do, we have to work, we have personal life, our analysis . . . why does it have to be so hard!".* Sometimes I didn't agree with what my supervisors said to me, it was difficult, many times they confronted me with mistakes I made and with things I had to work on my analysis. But I never felt judged.

For all this and more, dear Institute, I thank you for the opportunity to have received me with love and patience, for having seen me grow and mature. Now it is time to follow the path and be able to graduate to become an IPA (International Psychoanalytic Association) member and be a colleague of yours.

Warmly,

— Susana Maldonado Ponce

# 22 A letter to Institut de Psychanalyse de Montréal, Canada (1969)

## Nathalie Bissonnette

In Quebec, Canada, there are two separate Psychoanalytic Training Institute. Both are situated in the city of Montreal in the same building. One is a French speaking Training Institute based on the French psychoanalytic model. The other one is an English-speaking Training Institute, based on the Eitingon psychoanalytic model.

I am a French speaking Quebecoise. I decided to send my application to the "Institut de Psychanalyse de Montréal", the French side (because I speak French), without knowing the difference between either training models at the time. I was accepted during COVID's first wave of the pandemic catastrophe. I had three screening interviews with different Training Analysts. I remember my first interview: the Training Analyst telling me, that it was his first time to conduct a Zoom meeting (we did not know Zoom before COVID) and his first as a Training Analyst. It made me feel less like a candidate and more like a valued human being with the same anxieties, the same beginnings, the same unknown.

As you know in the French model, personal analysis is completely separated from the Training Institute and the Training Analysts. We have a four-year study program to go through. Three years are solely dedicated on Freud's writings and another year is used to teach the post Freudian like: Bion, Ferenczi, Aulagnier, Anzieu, Green, Lacan, Laplanche, The Middle Group, to name just a few.

The candidates are part of an open group which means that candidates are welcomed each year. It does create a different group dynamic. Conflicts and dissensions arise as well as great encounters. We must "attach and separate" every year, keeping us in a constant flux of uncertainties, like in an analysis. The regressions are frequent. The training, a constant source of analysis on the couch. As of today, we are a group of 14 candidates at different stages of training.

The Société Psychanalytique de Montréal has now less and less analysts. It feels like we can see each candidate that we crossed paths with, every month, even when they are done with the curriculum. I personally don't see a real difference between an open or closed group. Candidates come and go between other groups too, in other seminars. We can join in any seminar that welcomes new analysts.

DOI: 10.4324/9781003465409-22

*Candidates participate in debates during the once-a-month Scientific Con-
ferences, they are encouraged to write in the Bulletin, published three times
a year, under the auspices of the Société Psychanalytique de Montréal, the
French section of the Canadian Psychoanalytic Society. We are also encouraged to speak up whenever we have grievances. In addition, we have an
appointed mentor (another Training Analyst) that we can meet on a volunteer
basis. The mentor is a person with whom we discuss our training, our disappointments, hopes and grievances that arise within our group and with our
supervisors. He or she acts as a go between the candidate, the supervisor, and
the Training Committee.*

*We are also encouraged to start the controlled cases as soon as we feel
ready. That does not mean that it will count though. Sometimes, a candidate
must be supervised for a nonspecific period before he is approved for a controlled case. That was my condition for acceptance: to be supervised for a
controlled case that would not be part of the three controlled cases required
before we can proceed with application to become a member of the Société.*

———

Dear Institute,

One of the biggest challenges so far, is to tame the fact that psychoanalysis
is not what I thought it would be. It is not based on a scientific methodology,
and we are not taught current psychoanalysis trends. We are taught Freud.

I have always known that the common factor in all psychotherapies is
the quality of the relationship. The studies have all demonstrated this. For all
approaches, including psychoanalysis. I have explored all approaches; I have
been supervised in all approaches. For supervision, it's the same thing: the
dyad is the guarantor or not, of the learner's learning. But now I am learning that the quality of the relationship, in psychoanalysis, could be seen as
"negative transference" and we don't need to adjust nor adapt.

Since my acceptance, I have been able to observe several topics worthy
of further study: my entry during the pandemic, group processes, past dyads,
a beginning supervision of control cases and supervision for more difficult
cases. I was able to appreciate the quality of the course instructors and teachers I met with, both alone and in groups. I recognize the value of the teaching,
the richness of the sharing. However, I still feel like an outsider, despite all my
efforts to integrate, I keep coming up against an invisible membrane. I surely
would have appreciated a better integration process. Is it the homogeneity
of the group's clinical training? Is it the language, the words used in which
I no longer find myself? Is it my own issues that are being replayed? Is it the
apparent non-directionality that makes me feel like a ship without a captain?

Every educational institution brings its own color. I have experienced very
directive environments, sometimes too much so. I have also known environments that were too "loose", that lacked a long-term vision. I see you, dear

Institute, as an ambivalent environment, "loose" on the surface, but deep down, it seems rigid and non-inclusive, which can scare away those who don't say the right words, those who don't follow the line of the party in power.

I was selected but with catch-up criteria as you know. Yet no one could explain to me why I didn't fit in as is. I came from a "different" theoretical approach. I was not allowed to have two control cases at the same time. I was asked to do more without really bothering to contact my past supervisors or simply asking me how I worked. Getting closer to my world. Yet I thought I understood that psychoanalysis is at the heart of this: approaching another world. I understood afterwards that being educated in the land of CBT is very pejorative. And yet I have been working with transference and countertransference for years with treatment plans. I turned to you, dear Institute, precisely to be better equipped to deal with the unconscious and the treatment plan.

Dear Institute, here is an example from a CBT treatment manual:[1]

> The methodology of the clinician is not the aim of psychotherapy . . . What needs to be guarded against is a clinician forgetting the patient's stated goals and allowing the methods or theories of treatment to gradually shift the treatment contract and the aim of the therapy from what the patient was seeking, to something that serves the clinicians preferred theories or techniques.
> The goals sought for most patients:
>
> - hope to change
> - hope of proving that no one can change them
> - desire to reduce or stop the suffering
> - desire to be comforted while retaining their defining suffering
> - desire for a change of perspective
> - desire to avoid "central issues", to make modest gains with certain symptoms.

Psychoanalysis, on the other hand, teaches us to move away from the representation of purpose, from goals, to allow the being to emerge. Candidates are asked to suspend their own goals such as having a control case, wanting to cure or to help, wanting to teach or accompany, wanting to relieve patient's sufferings. I am asking you, dear Institute, how is that possible? Personally, I find that different approaches would benefit from talking to each other and benefit from looking for common spaces rather than focusing on the differences.

Organizational psychology teaches certain basics about managing organizations: planning, organizing, controlling. Dear Institute, why did you choose to only deal with the "control" part? I don't understand that the very notions of plans, planning, organizing are off-putting for an analyst when it's all about "framework", "holding", "interpretation", etc. I also wish that the curriculum would be given in order, presenting each text according to Freud's train of thought and not according to teacher's availability and interest. Maybe, if the teachers were paid, the pay would serve as an incentive to give good, valuable teaching format. I remember being very frustrated when given to read on the "Unconscious" before reading about "Repression" for example or having read *Interpretation of Dreams* after more than six months of Freud's material. For me, that does not make any sense.

Dear Institute, at one point we, as a clinical community, we will have to start building bridges between approaches. The risk of analysis disappearing is very real. If I, who come from another approach, who have chosen to train in analysis, cannot find my way around, how can we expect other colleagues to want to undertake such a training?

Becoming an analyst has been a "saut de l'ange" for me. A fellow candidate even said that he would never undertake a training in another approach than psychodynamic. I felt like if I was "jumping into the unknown". Before I was accepted, before I applied, I could describe myself as a seasoned CBT clinician, EMDR trained, specialized with PTSD veterans. But that was before. There is a now. There will probably be an after since I am in mid-training. I would just like to say that I went from a "knowing-specialist" posture to feeling like a rookie "lost in translation", lost in training, lost like a child.

I thought I was joining a contemporary psychoanalytic Training Institute like the other ones in North America. Instead, I have learned that there is dissension, rivalry between psychoanalysis schools in North America. There is no such thing in CBT. The trainings just adds on with the scientific data if proven to be reliable. I did not know that what I had learned about attachment for example or how to come up with a diagnosis would become irrelevant in psychoanalysis training. Why is that?

I view psychoanalytic training as a shedding process. You must "let go". Forget about DSM and treatment plans. Letting go of a skin without being able to grow one back. It hurts. It is demanding emotionally, financially, and on the family. I fear that I could lose some of my professional self in that process of "forgetting". Is that what is required of candidates? What if I find myself not being able to provide a simple treatment plan in a few years? What if I forget the techniques that took me years to build on? Why am I not able to provide space for these thoughts within my group of peer-candidates? Why am I afraid of being analyzed for my choices of clinical practice like if I had done something wrong?

Dear Institute, I have to say I wish I would have been more prepared. I say this as a warning maybe, a "en garde" for future candidates that are as green as we can be. I probably have my part in that play. But I also think that you could have one too. It takes more efforts to accompany someone who does not know psychoanalytic institutions. I knew I wanted to learn a new method just like Irvine Yalom suggested. The more we know, the better we become not the more we know, the more corrupt we can be . . .

Freud was a stranger to me. I wish now, looking back, that I would have read some basic books like: "Lire Freud" de Jean-Michel Quinodoz (Reading Freud)[2] and the "Manuel de psychologie et de psychopathologie clinique générale" de René Roussillon[3] (The not yet translated Handbook of Psychology and General Clinical Psychopathology). I was fortunate enough to come across these two books when I questioned my fellow candidates on their best readings. Dear Institute, why did it not come from you? It took two years before I got my way around. I feel a little angry, not well accompanied for the transition. I think I sometime start to agree with one of the harshest critics against psychoanalysis as it is an approach that is elitist, not well enough researched as to how to teach it.

Dear Institute, are you sure about the three-year program solely on Freud? I am afraid it will come as a religion. We must believe. Freud has been criticized before. Can the candidates do so as well without being told to read first and then criticize? Can we be provided with a safe space to discuss a topic without being scolded like children? I remember a fellow candidate who left after trying to discuss the unconscious from a neuroscience point of view. Can we allow this to happen in a contemporary training Institute?

And can I suggest again to give the texts to read in an order that makes sense? It is difficult to understand why we were taught a text on *Witt* before having read *The Interpretation of Dreams* for example. I think that, maybe, since the teachers are not paid, it becomes obviously difficult to ask them for specifics in the program but then, can we (the candidates) ask for more professionalism from our Institute? I am afraid that when I go to some conferences World Wide, that I won't be prepared.

Dear Institute, thinking back, I must have gone through a denying process (even though I was told) that I would have to do some additional supervisory time. I feel like if I did not have what it takes to become an analyst although I had spent numerous years on a couch. You say that a candidate who comes from a background like mine will be asked to do more supervisory time than a candidate who is familiar with the psychoanalytic thinking. At first it would appear logical to do so, but in practice, it must be very difficult to assess. What are your exact criteria? Although I had had numerous dialectic supervisors during my career (25 years plus), it did not count. It is very difficult to assess and compare training. I had to accept the challenge and the regression that goes with it, as part of my path. To this day I can't give a general direction or rule of thumb as to how you go from a supervised controlled case that does not count for your training, to a controlled case that counts. Numbers or figures are out of that equation, and it still very frustrating for me.

Dear Institute, I am afraid.

You know that it is hard to offer psychoanalysis to potential analysands. Most of our patients are asking for relief, for the symptoms to disappear. Most can't sustain three times a week. It is a fact that psychoanalysis is not seen as a cure. So tell me, dear Institute, tell me what should I say to patients because I am running out of words.

This critical and sometimes condescending attitude towards the various other schools of thought in psychology cannot encourage the transmission of psychoanalysis in our societies. I had read about it. Now I can say that it is true. I think that it creates and perpetuates a schism from which psychoanalysis does not emerge victorious these days. Here in my French-Canadian town, Montreal, psychoanalysts are a dying breed, like I said earlier. I think that having intervision (supervision within peers) would allow a pooling of resources. I have not seen invitations sent to other types of clinicians or researchers as of yet.

Dear Institute, I stop counting the times that I thought "I quit, this is it!"

I remember times where I would argue my case with my supervisor, in an absolute, totally, regressive state. During this whole process, I sure felt as a "rotten", bad little girl. Truth be told, I thought my supervisor was very supportive in her special way of listening to my complaints. I knew she could not decide all by herself. It took a nearly two years before I was authorized to work on a controlled case that would count towards my being as a psychoanalyst. My supervisor presented my previous cases to "Le Comité de l'Enseignement" (The Committee on Education) and gave them proof of life. The proof that I understood the difference between psychoanalysis and other approaches. The proof, if there is such a thing, that I knew what could be analyzed as part of a transference process and what could not be.

What if I had known all of this before I decided to get on with the program? And how could I have known? Let's face it, nothing can really prepare us for that task, just like in analysis. I consider myself lucky to have been able to choose my analyst and to choose my supervisor. Like Allanah Furlong[4] said: "lucky . . . to have been able to freely follow the folly of my idealization and fixation with someone who accepted to be "used" by me" in a Winnicottian and a Roussillon sense".

Nevertheless, I still wonder if I could have been better accompanied during the transition. I wish that I could have had the opportunity to present myself to the Committee and not to be treated solely based on the fact that I was trained as a CBT practitioner. After all, I had been on a couch for quite a while before I applied. I am pretty sure that no one in the Committee, nor my supervisor, knows exactly what CBT or any other approaches or techniques entails. We are told, as Candidate, to suspend our judgement towards Freud's writing under the pretext of "you cannot criticize unless you have read and know what you are talking about". I wish the same would have applied in the case of CBT, intersubjective, humanistic, or medical background.

This enterprise, "becoming a psychoanalyst", is not experienced as an amalgam, a fusion with other clinical approaches. It is rather like a wrench. The old knowledge, the lived, the known, the useful for the insurance companies or the third-party payers, becomes less and less accessible. An erasure is taking place. My task is that of separation, of separating the bodies, of making a new skin. A skin of my own. Not that of Freud and his followers, not that of my analyst, not that of my supervisor. One day, I wrote a short poem (Bissonnette, 2022). I had a dream following a discussion about the place of the body in analysis. This text was then published in the Bulletin, and I share it with you here:

*Perched high*
*My village of hills*
*And my bedroom*
*I woke up*
*In hollow*
*A cry, from the dream*
*Open your door for me*
*My beautiful love, my truth*
*I received in the morning*
*Psyche fainted*
*In the arms of Soma*
*Tired*
*Defeated*
*Hair in battle*
*Romeo and Juliet*
*Coming from afar*
*From adolescence*
*Like us*
*Drifting from river to river*
*Like us, on the couch*
*Stranded on the couch*
*Breath to take again*
*Their hands seek each other*
*Soma is worried*
*Do not shake me, I am full of tears*
*Weft to weave, words of rain*
*Rest hoped for*
*Like a bush under the snow*
*I observe like the one before me*
*The awakening of Psyche*
*Clings to the face of Soma*
*Autumn morning nimbed by the purple sunrise*
*Witnesses of the embrace*
*I*
*Breathe*
*They leave, gone*

*Like us*
*Creators*
*(October 2021)*


Dear Institute, to this day, I don't know what kind of analyst I will be . . . probably a little more interventionist than others, I suppose. Or maybe I'll be a life-long candidate . . . someone who refuses to be part of an Institute . . . Unless I submit on the surface and then develop my own practice, my own style?

But I know of no other training institute where clinical issues are discussed in sometimes medical, social, philosophical, phenomenological terms and in a literary language of its own. That is why I am still pursuing this training: I know that nowhere else is there such a learning experience!

Food for thought . . . like I said: oscillating.

Let us not forget that Homo omini lupus est ("Man is a wolf to another man").

— Nathalie Bissonnette


## Notes

1 Leeds, A. M. (2009). *A guide to the standard EMDR protocols for clinicians, supervisors, and consultants* (pp. 71–72). Springer Publishing Company.
2 Quinodoz, J. (2004). *Lire Freud*. PUF.
3 Roussillon, R. (2018). *Manuel de psychologie et de psychopathologie clinique générale*. Elsevier Masson.
4 Furlong, A. (2020). *Dear candidate: Analysts from around the world offer personal reflections on psychoanalytic training, education and the profession* (F. Busch, Ed., pp. 73–75). Routledge.

# 23 A letter to Sociedad Psicoanalítica de México, Mexico City (1972)

*Erika Lepiavka*

*The Psychoanalytic Society of Mexico is first and foremost, a community. September 19th, 2017, was a before and after moment. The earth shook with tremor rendering central Mexico into chaos. Familiar areas became ghastly. Our premises with lovely views to Parque México, suddenly became part of a ground zero area. The shadow of the object was unseen, because the object had fallen to the ground, taking over the air we were breathing. In the middle of the anxieties that arise in such destruction, the members of our Institute and Society came together as a solid group. We joined our forces to fight the tragedy that surrounded us as citizens with psychoanalytic thought, sharing the desire to help and care for others. We learned our limits and our potential. We went into disaster zones, while we took care of each other, physically and mentally. We learned from other disciplines, thanks to the previous links our society had with associations that are specialized in handling these crises. We mourned for what was gone. We helped each other in the restoration of our own thinking apparatus.*

*Weeks into this experience brought back to me a memory from when I was in the first years of elementary school. During those days the Mexican Secretariat of Education (Secretaría de Educación Pública) gave textbooks to all its students across the country. These books often talked about "your community". Growing up in a place where the streets were dangerous and no place to play in, I often wondered what the word community even meant. It was after this 2017 "season in hell"[1] that the estrangement towards the word community was replaced by its meaning.*

*I will now tell you a little bit about how the Institute of Psychoanalysis[2] where I train became what it is today. Sociedad Psicoanalítica de México was founded in 1972 as a Study Group. While its roots date back to 1944, it started in the seventies with what was then a bold proposal: to make psychoanalytic training available to non-medical healthcare providers. In the core of its identity lies its boldness. It was founded by a generation of refugees who settled in Mexico and later traveled across the American continent to become IPA Psychoanalysts. It took decades of fighting for its honour that finally gained its recognition as an IPA Component Society in 2007. During*

DOI: 10.4324/9781003465409-23

the 47th IPA Congress in Mexico in 2011, it was casually nick-named the society of the youth. Its commitment to the surrounding community is explicit. It has pursued through decades to make psychoanalysis available to the general population. It aims towards innovation while it honours the classics. Its innovative qualities go along with its loyalty to the truth. I am referring to what Anna Freud (1968) described as the essential trait to becoming a real psychoanalyst "A great appreciation for truth, personal truth and scientific truth". Its plurality of thought is maintained by a strong ideal of respect to our differences. Institute and Society are a team, much like its members. We care for each other, strive to maintain respect above all, and function as a psychoanalytic community through the hardships (and the delights) of life.

To this date, our premises on Parque México remain uninhabitable. Its community maintains itself strong, active and very much alive. The debate resonates through past, present and future generations.

The views expressed come from my own voice, which is often heard in my consulting room. This quiet and special spot was found in the days following the 2017 earthquake, thanks to the generosity of one of my colleagues. This place became a dream amid a nightmare. A spot finally opened for me in this building in November of 2020. In the middle of the pandemic, I remembered Roberto Gaitan's[3] words; you pay for your admission interviews, and that is your bet. I have been betting ever since. I have lost, and I have won. **And I get by, with a little help from my friends.**[4]

—

Dear Institute,

It has been two and a half years since I took my last seminars with you. We said, "*see you soon*", in February of 2022. A few weeks later, the state of sanitary emergency was declared due to the new Coronavirus pandemic. Ever since, I have been faced with the challenges of keeping my practice alive without the container your seminars gave shape to.

The first days of 2020 seemed full of promise, after finally reaching the goal that seemed impossible so many times; the completion of a demanding six-year seminar program. "*What once seemed like a summit, is now the ground*", said one of our professors during our last class. Our group was sad to leave seminars, "*a uno le duele lo que fue bueno*",[5] Carlino[6] said to us. And so, between the feelings of mourning and fulfillment, our transformed consulting rooms became deserted. The first case of Coronavirus was detected in Mexico on the 27th of February of 2020.

The previous year had been one with different personal losses, which had been more bearable in your presence, dear Institute. Seminars were never easy, but they always gave me in return as much as I put into them. *Giving and receiving,* was the name of the game. A game we played with passion and dedication, like an Olympic sport. We had reached the last game, and personal grief that had been in motion until March 2020, suddenly stood still, in a quarantined world.

I had been lucky enough to take seminars and supervise cases with Carlino, a pioneer in what he and a group of colleagues named *Distance Analysis* at some point between 2005 and 2011. During my seminar years, I was confronted with the possibility of turning the virtual space into an analytic space. I had read Carlino's book (2010) and practiced his teachings in different settings (for example, when my consulting room was unreachable after the 2017 earthquake, or when a patient migrated). My personal paradigm on remote sessions had been shaken long before the pandemic forced us all to move into the virtual space. In this sense, I felt I had an advantage. In the absence of seminars, however, I felt terribly alone.

I started my training some days late due to being sick with Influenza. When I emailed my professors to ask about the reading for the classes I had missed, I remember receiving one particular response—"*what matters to me is that you recover*". This was Luisa Rossi,[7] our soon-to-be Institute Director.

The mission was uphill—two years for a master's degree in Psychoanalytic Psychotherapy, plus one year for a Specialty Degree, and at least three more of *la formación propiamente dicha* (the psychoanalytic training properly speaking, which is IPA approved). Four hundred hours of supervision or control analysis, with five different supervisors and different criteria. Personal analysis is essential at all stages of this process. I began my training with a clinical background in Psychology and field work in community settings. It was after my first semester that I found myself standing on the border of Tijuana and San Diego, thinking why this uncanny place existed. This was the first time I found myself applying psychoanalytic concepts to the context that surrounded me. I thought this could be the subject of my first paper presentation. It didn't happen. The question has remained, nonetheless. It took me one semester in your program for me to dive into a question I am still looking for answers to, dear Institute.

Training to become a psychoanalyst really was an avalanche; of thought, discovery, confrontation, and all the stages one is immersed during this venture. I had my energy devoted to seminars, the intense reading load, the papers to be presented, the cases to work through. During these years, we navigated different universes: Freud's Vienna, the Salpêtrière, Clark University, Freud's London. Mrs. Klein came along and took us on another dimension. At this point, many were already on our boat: Mrs. Horney, Mr. Fenichel, Mr. Abraham, Mrs. Anna Freud, Mrs. Mahler, Mr. Winnicott, Mr. Ramírez. But it was Mrs. Klein who broke my scheme in an *aprés-coup* fashion. During a seminar on Psychoanalytic Technique (some years after digesting Object Relations Theory), I found myself writing my response to Bion's Differentiation of the Psychotic from the Non-Psychotic Personalities (1957), "It seems to me, like I need to second-think Melanie Klein's theory". Soon after, Mr. Racker, Mrs. Bick, Mr. Rosenfeld (both of them), Mrs. and Mr. Baranger, Mrs. Bleichmar, Mr. Searles, Mr. Resnik would step onto the boat, to break some more schemes. Mr. Rousillon, Mr. Anzieu, Mr. Ferro—the list is endless.

It was thanks to the earlier strict teaching of Alejandro Beltrán[8] that I was able to understand the inner workings of the mind as splits, as bits and pieces. Thank you, dear Comrade, for diving me into Mrs. Klein's brilliance. Training requires us to face the most unpleasant parts of humankind. It makes us go through constant regressions; it tests our limits. Training is a test on memory, capacity for, and appreciation of knowledge. At the Institute of Psychoanalysis of Sociedad Psicoanalítica de México, the *Rotatorios clínicos* (Rotary Clinical Seminars), are composed of a proliferous clinical history, a treatment summary, three psychoanalytic case formulations and two sessions presented along with one Training Analyst who changes every two weeks. At least one scientific paper is required per semester, which is to be presented in a Congress format. Each semester is composed by four to six seminars. One must demonstrate during this time that one can conduct oneself as a psychoanalyst. You may be regressed, but you must relate to others as the adult you are. A solid Ethics Committee makes sure we demonstrate we have what is needed to be analysts in training.

During our last toast, the candidates finishing seminars were asked by Carlino to give a speech. Although I tried to hide, one of my professors spotted and encouraged me. I was terribly nervous. What does one say to the entire Institute, on the last toast as a candidate? I said what was in my heart: *"This has become an object to me, and I wonder what I will do without it!"*

It is now when I would like to speak of a theory I have developed ever since. In order for me to tell this theory, I would like to speak of a latter experience. I recently had the honour of being part of the jury for an international writing award on psychoanalysis. As I read these carefully selected finalist papers, I noticed myself being overcritical of them. I gave these articles some time to rest, and in the meantime, I realized: I am being too *demanding,* or more precisely, in Spanish, *exigente.* It was at this point, in the middle of 2022, that it became clear to me; the seminars have remained inside my mind for more than two years. My psychoanalytic brothers and sisters had become objects themselves, along with my professors. They have kept on arguing, pointing out, maintained rigor in the way I work with my patients. My theory is, dear Institute, that what we have is a bond. And it is that bond that shapes me, every day.

I have been completing my supervision cases required by my training program to be able to obtain the Psychoanalyst diploma by the International Psychoanalytical Association. I supervise cases with Doctor Kiyotaka Osawa, an analyst whose technique I describe as 'Kyionian', but I am certain he could describe himself as either; a modern Freudian, a Bionian, a neo-bionan, a grossteinian, a follower of Bollas and Ogden, and an applier of Zen Buddhism on his style of interpreting. Dr. Osawa, *Kiyo,* as I call him, introduced to me his concept of *mental quarantine* in the summer of 2020. At the beginning of confinement, when I asked him how he was, he said, *I feel challenged. It is in these times when I feel most energized.* It was through phone sessions that Kiyotaka held me during the anguishes of being an analyst in training during a pandemic. There is something special and unique about speaking to a survivor of the Second World War.

In Spanish, *formar* means to give shape to. We rarely call it "entrenami-ento" (training). *Formación psicoanalítica* is the usual term. You have given shape to the clinician within me. And in this process, you have allowed me to maintain my essence. **Thank you, dear Institute, for not being vertical, nor horizontal.** I am not sure what the number is, what angle would it be, but you allow enough pendant for boundaries to be understood, hierarchies to be respected, while inviting dialogue and constant questioning, enabling creativity and stimulating psychoanalytic thought. You have found a sort of *sana distancia* or healthy distance, that has allowed me to grow psychically while respecting the limits of the outer world.

We had ups and downs, dear Institute. I am grateful for having a couch on which I felt free to vent on the many frustrations imposed by the process of training. I was able to regress freely and complain like a teenager, as a child throwing a tantrum, or even a crying baby. Thank you, dear Analyst, for hold-ing and handling this. The ups were good; our local congresses, Perú, Bue-nos Aires, London, New York. The happiness after leaving a case presentation feeling nourished with ideas of a whole group of analysts in training from dif-ferent stages of it. Presenting a paper and going back home to read your notes because you got bright, refreshing feedback. Laughing at some silly joke in the middle of a seminar. Seeing colleagues and friends; associating together as peers, creating chains of thought. And then, there were more lows. As any idealized object, you went into the opposite direction many times. Thank you, dear Analyst, for noting this whenever it was needed. Then times got worse: we lost our premises facing Parque México. To this day, it saddens me when I pass by the park on the way to my consulting room and I see the remains of our building. Even so, this never stopped us. From venue to venue, we found a way to meet and keep thinking when we needed it the most.

*Constancy, no matter what*, is a sort of motto I have learned from one of my supervisors. I believe that as an Institute, you have shown that attitude. Rain or shine, your seminars take place, dear Institute. Rain or shine, the training must go on. Constancy, because a constant object is what a patient needs.

This letter is mostly meant to thank you, dear Institute. After two and a half years of distance, I have had the chance to digest the intense travesty of con-cepts we navigated. I have gone through all the states of mourning for your seminars. However, it has been a long time since I passed the angry phase of mourning. It is in this distance, that I want to thank you. And I do warn you, dear reader, this list might be long.

Thank you, dear Institute, for seeing potential in me. Thank you for point-ing out my flaws when it was needed, and for doing so in a safe space. Thank you for demanding so much form me, that I now know the ground I step on is steady, strong, and genuine. Thank you, dear Institute, for your trust in me. Thank you for being critical of me. Thank you for being supportive of me. I have been asked to be critical towards you in this letter. However, I must decline this tempting invitation. Thank you, dear Institute, for showing me the difference between the public and the private. My memories of you are predominantly positive. As an object relation, dear Institute, you are a total one. And in your totality, you have been good-enough. You are not perfect, as nothing is. *There is beauty in imperfection*, Kiyotaka would say.

I write to you now, dear Institute, not only as a graduate of your seminars that fulfills hours of supervisions, but also as IPSO President-Elect. And so now I thank you, *querido Instituto*, for always making space for IPSO. Thank you for preparing and encouraging us to participate in national and international congresses, for allowing us to write freely, and for always giving me space to interrupt your seminars with IPSO announcements. You were there, dear Institute, since the first time I presented in our IPSO/IPA Buenos Aires Congress on Intimacy. You were there, when I presented at FEPAL/OCAL's Congress in Lima, *Construcciones y Deconstrucciones*. You were there, when I presented in London, on *The Feminine*. You were there, in this year's EPF Congress, *Ideals*. You were everywhere, for our latest FEPAL Congress, *Transitoriedades e incertezas,* in a virtual yet warm Mexico. You are always there, dear Institute. You are part of my self.

It is with this distance that I write to you, dear Institute. You have shown me support like no other academic frame has. It is at this moment in time that I write—September 2022—that the feelings of gratitude and admiration persist towards you. I miss you, sometimes. And when I say sometimes, it's because I know you're there, one text message away. And you are there many times a week in the spaces that have kept me afloat as an analyst in training through a pandemic, my analyst, Marina, and my supervisor, Kiyo. This is to them, and to Ricardo Carlino. Carlino, thank you for reminding me after the 2017 earthquake that *crisis means opportunity.* Thank you for in April 2020, when I asked you how you were, you said in an enthusiastic tone "¡Bien! ¡Estamos vivos!" (Doing well! We are alive!). Thank you for calling me authentic when I was unsure of myself and my future. Kiyo, thank you for pointing psychoanalytic cracks with your judo-skills and fearless attitude. Marina, *gracias*.

Thank you, to all of my professors who have now become objects of my inner world. You are still there, challenging me, constantly helping me grow. You are present, dear Institute, through my colleagues who are also my friends, with whom the psychoanalytic debate continues. So many characters have gotten on board of this boat called *la formación psicoanalítica,* which is always symbolically laying in Parque México. The list of characters is long, and the boat is fascinating. The memories and faces keep springing up in my mind. Thank you, to my symbolic brothers and sisters, who have traversed this ocean of psychoanalytic waves along with me. Thank you, dear Rosalba,[9] for being the role model this woman will always need.

Finally, thank you, dear Institute, for enabling me to believe I could run for IPSO President. Thank you for your support function, and for the trust you put in my hands for such role. I hope to always be up to the very high standards you raise.

*Con cariño,*

— Erika Lepiavka

## Notes

1 To quote Rimbaud's *Une saison en enfer.*
2 Instituto de Estudios de Posgrado en Psicoanálisis y Psicoterapia S.C. is our Institute's full name.
3 Dr. Roberto Gaitán, Institute Director from 1991 until his premature death in 2017.
4 Lennon, P. McCartney, 1967.
5 'One aches for what was good'.
6 Ricardo Carlino MD. Psychiatrist. Psychoanalyst. Full Member Asocaición Psicoanalítica de Buenos Aires (APdeBA). Supervisor, Professor and Full Member of Sociedad Psicoanlítica de México (SPM).
7 Dr. Luisa Rossi, Training Analyst and Institute Director.
8 Dr. Alejandro Beltrán, President of the Psychoanalytic Society of Mexico.
9 Dr. Rosalba Bueno, Institute Director and Chair of the Ethics Committee.

# 24 A letter to the Australian Psychoanalytic Society, Sydney (1973)

*Leticia Aydos*

*The Australian Psychoanalytic Society (APAS) history is intwined with the Australian tale of distance, compulsory or otherwise war-tinged migration as well as growth borne out of the exquisite combination between grief, loss and opportunity (Boots 2010). Although an incipient interest in psychoanalysis from as far as 1911 was indeed seen, it was not until 1940 with the arrival of Clara Geroe to Melbourne that the first Psychoanalytic Institute was formed. Clara was a Hungarian psychoanalyst trained in Budapest and was escaping WWII. She was appointed as a training analyst by the British Psychoanalytic Society and the Institute in Melbourne functioned as a branch to the British Society. Development progressed slowly, making use of creativity, interdisciplinary connections and outreach activities. The Australian Society became a Component Society in 1973. With the assistance from IPA visiting committees the current structure we nowadays have, of a unified society with three branches, Sydney, Melbourne and Adelaide, prevailed. European arrivals revived the analytic spirit in Australia— commemorations to Neville and Joan Symington in acknowledgement of their immensurable contributions have been had or are underway. Also, the Society this year will commemorate its 50th Anniversary—there is a vibrancy to the group which feels linked to celebrating the arduous trajectory between challenging beginnings to a thriving community—Australian, after all.*

*Currently, training with APAS is in accordance to IPA requirements.*

- *A first-year infant observation with weekly visits and weekly seminars is a requirements for all candidates.*
- *Candidates are asked to see two cases with a duration of two years each.*
- *Attendance to Theoretical and Clinical seminars are for three and four years, respectively.*
- *Candidates are expected to attend to interstate weekends occurring three times a year in Melbourne, Sydney and Adelaide.*
- *A research project is to be completed by candidates during their training.*

—

DOI: 10.4324/9781003465409-24

Now, to the Dear Institute of which I am a candidate, here I speak:

> In his late work, Bion pictures the self as what might poetically be called 'a colony of souls'. One cannot imagine all the participants of this colony ever being integrated; rather, what is important is making contact and communicating across time and space with the myriad characters and energies that proliferate and gain access to consciousness. In this model, the self has a kind of kaleidoscopic complexity as an evolving process.
>
> —J Eaton in *Building a Floor for Experience (Eaton, 2015)*

Amidst many other life experiences and connections, this quote moved a desire to engage in analytic training into an action that involved applying for training and then becoming a candidate. I have since been discovering the analytic village where I now inhabit. The quote above I believe can be applied to the training ambience. Once a child growing in a military dictatorship, I have been cautious of totalitarian views. I have had the benefit of parents who did not conform and have always left an open channel with us children. This quote conveys to me a deep form of openness and coherence. Something I would very much like to embark upon and explore. Starting analytic training has been a complex experience, such as growing up. Similar to my experience at home, here I feel there is a channel open between you and me.

When a woman is pregnant with their first child it is indeed so difficult to explain to her what is to come, perhaps because it is an experience that is unique for each person. There is a proportion of the experience, however, that is rather universal. Possibly, no one would prefer to tell such rough truths to the poor pregnant lady. Imagine saying to her "well, darling, this will be like taking an international flight across a few many time-zones every second or, if you are lucky, third day . . ." As I was approaching the decision to enter training and communicated my thoughts to your member analysts, I was often met with an enigmatic expression in their faces. I have now been able to better interpret the expression as: "this will be like taking an international flight across many time-zones every second or, if you are lucky, third day . . ." which they seemed disinclined to tell me directly in case I rushed to take a morning-after-pill. This was alongside a delight to hear I was carrying a growing life in my mind. My experience was of a warm, alive, welcoming and facilitating process.

Some people have braved to tell me about certain aspects of the process. I think they did this out of conscientiousness and a sense of ethics. One of them drew me a detailed calculation as to how much, realistically, training would cost. As she spoke, I knew this was the truth and knew I did not want to know this truth. I then commented that this calculation did not apply to me so much because I only worked part time. The same knowing voice, the one who knew there was truth there, echoed in my mind "and time?" She was correct in many accounts. Another person yet, referred to the experience of training as "very intense, demanding, verging traumatic". I then asked him whether he felt it was even worth the effort given they felt traumatised. He then said, "I said *verging* traumatic". One will only hear what one wants to hear and how one wants to hear it. I was not impressed with either view at the time. It was possible for me to come to other members of the village and speak, hear their perspectives and make up my own mind. This is what I say to you, in this village of yours, there is a channel open to the children and I believe strongly this to be essential.

During this decision-making time, there was a loss by suicide in the Society, by one of the younger members. I knew this person to some degree due to professional affiliations. This loss raised questions of whether this village was good, safe, whether it protected the children well or not, whether it taught the children how to look after themselves. Well, you know, I put the question to some of your most senior members. I was met with openness and humble humanness, similar to what I received as a child all the way back to the home I come from. I witnessed how deeply touched by this tragedy the village members really were. Dear Institute, here there is a small analytic family where things can become rather tight for all involved. Everyone knows one another rather well. Say the good friend you made in the beginning of training: their analyst could (very) easily also be theirs or be your supervisor and vice-versa. Supervisors may know you from other walks of life. They may be an analytic sibling. In my view, this can become so claustrophobic that the only way out is to become bold, embrace oneself and brace forward. Perhaps not everyone can manage this feat.

Another complication is, as you know, there are not many people to train candidates— training analysts and non-training analysts seem to be spread thinly on the ground, working very hard. There have been bitter losses of senior analysts due to rapidly progressing health events. A never-ending wave of retirements. People seem to have found ways to manage: there is a movement to connect the various branches of training across states to make for better opportunities of entry and connection for all. International connections are also encouraged and facilitated; a refreshing positive outcome born out of a problem. Having a supervisor who is outside the analytic village is arguably an element of vital importance during analytic training. More naturally the topic in supervision becomes psychoanalysis. This is in opposition to getting caught in between parents who could be disagreeing or, worse, fighting due to differences in opinion, in personal style and adherence to local factions. Struggles are inherent, as it seems, to analytic societies. An outsider is in a privileged and neutral position in order to help.

Institute, now I am here, and I have made an interesting observation while in training: an overwhelming sense of mental tiredness after a string of activities. This I have coined to myself as "psychoanalytic tiredness". In this community there is an activity that occurs three times a year called Interstate Weekends—this you would know very well. Our training bodies in Sydney,

Melbourne and Adelaide host a weekend once a year. Local analysts work hard organising activities for the day which might include readings, discussions as well as sections of infant observation and clinical case discussions when we are divided into smaller groups. This is anticipated by us candidates with eagerness, especially after the long isolating experience during the pandemic years. I have not yet discovered who came up with this idea originally, it is brilliant and participating in it has been a challenge. At the end of Saturday, which is always the busiest day with morning and afternoon activities occurring, there is a sense I experienced of a mushy brain, or a brain that has paled and is not functioning. There is little capacity for interactions, social talks or anything really. One fellow candidate said, "my brain hurts". Now having a second look, perhaps pain is well suited to the situation as an analogy. The brilliant idea is so in many levels. In one level, it presents candidates to one another who are training interstate and therefore influenced by different currents. This is most enriching. In another level yet, it can illustrate to us candidates 'live' what analysts can get up to in their collective madness: this group of people who sit for hours pushing their minds to the edge of unknowing/existence in a very abstract manner reaching to one's own unconscious mind as well as the group's. It is addictive, no doubt. There is a hint of dopamine release to it, a thrill: connecting with others in a parallel form of existence. Let's hold hands and bungee jump! However, this is the actual part that's missing: the jumping. Forgetting there is also a body with needs, a need for movement. Sometimes getting out of the "mind" and moving is essential for life, it also moves the mind. I suppose here I am saying, my Institute, that I am concerned for the health of the village, as well as my own.

I have so far wondered whether this lack of movement that intrinsically seems to exist has been contributing in some way to the notorious troubles that take place inside societies. A group of people sitting for long periods of time and thinking deeply leads to many good things and . . . also trouble. Vascular issues are a fine example as people put on weight, enlarge their abdominal circumferences and slowly lose their executive function. No wonder reputable training analysts get into boundary breaches and worse at the end of their careers—according to what I have been taught in seminars. When I first heard about the realities of such violations, I experienced a sense of shock and fear . . . then, giving it more thought, my institute, it unfortunately made sense to me.

Before training I had a good exercise routine, my weight was within the healthy range, I was learning Yoga and how to play the guitar. Obediently to the class, one year on, I have stopped exercising and am now in the overweight section. I managed to, with white knuckles, hold on to the guitar classes. Oftentimes I described interpersonal exchanges in the context of training to my guitar teacher, only for him to say: "Leticia, drop out of this course, it will stifle your mind". He has later added "well, perhaps staying is the wiser position because you have your eyes on the prize". Yes, I say, the baby. I have since returned to a once-a-week exercise routine, am determined to increase this and return the weight back to normal. This was after a conversation with the same analyst who told me originally about financial costs. This time the talk revolved around maintaining good health in this most challenging and seated profession. This time I paid closer attention to her. Some truths are sobering, my Dear Institute.

Your members have also told me that the returns of embarking in this business could be in the realm of mind blowing. I can attest to this so far: I have made deep international connections back with my homeland as well as with around-the-globe candidates. This has been encouraged and nurtured by you. The International Psychoanalytic Association has, as an organisation, become aware of stagnation issues and that global, multicultural connections are a good antidote against it. This local village is following those international steps.

I was discussing the South American position as one of the strong epicentres of psychoanalytic development in the contemporary psychoanalytic landscape with one of your senior members. This is the land where I was borne . . . my shoulders dropped as did my face, "oh dear, why did I leave". As I became aware of my own display of emotion, I immediately apologised. The response I received was astounding, really, he said: "you know, Leticia, here in Australia we are used to people questioning their decision about here . . ." All corners of the Earth will have their wounds. I have mine; you have yours. It is humbling, though, to experience being taken in so openly even while demonstrating a certain degree of rejection. It was as if I was told "people question their 'being' in Australia, but now you *are* here, and we *do* take you".

In relation to the actual "work" of training, I have observed from various points of contact I am offered a "dance of infants" together with the trainers. I feel honoured by this opportunity. Perhaps the gratitude I am describing here is an earned one, a product from getting into scuffles with myself and others, only to come out the other way remembering the humanity of all involved. After all, all involved here are only humans.

— Leticia Aydos

# 25 A letter to Asociación Psicoanalítica de Buenos Aires, Argentina (1977)

*Marìa Florencia Biotti*

*At the end of 1977, APdeBA (Buenos Aires Psychoanalytical Association) was established in order to promote and develop Psychoanalysis as a science, as a method of treatment and as a way of research of mental processes.*

*Postgraduate training programs were developed there as an entity belonging to Medicine University (UBA).*

*APdeBA has a high international reputation and carries out different activities in a permanent atmosphere of theoretical-clinical exchange.*

*Since APdeBA had decided to support University Education, IUSAM (Mental Health University Institute) was created in 2005. IPA training in APdeBA depends on IUSAM.*

*Consequently, it is important to mention that with this creation APdeBA moved on toward a proposal articulation among Psychoanalysis, Mental Health and University training. Its purpose is to suitably accompany the change process that Psychoanalysis is going through and to be included in Society from the totality of the perspective of Mental Health problems.*

*Regarding requirements to graduate, you need to*

- *Do seminars. You have an evaluation at the end of each seminar (in general it is a written work).*
- *You have two supervisions of two years each one. The control cases must be high frequency cases. You can do two cases of adults or you can do one of them with a child (it was my choice).*
- *At the end you have to do an integrating work of the whole training which is evaluated for a jury of three senior analysts.*

—

## On my experience of becoming an analyst

I propose to reflect on the particular adventure shared by all of us who undertake and go through the experience of becoming an analyst.

DOI: 10.4324/9781003465409-25

I have an image, a common place in fairy tales. The protagonist comes out of the castle stripped off all his or her real attributes. Now he or she has only a kind of broomstick from which hangs a rag bag with certain indispensable elements and then, he or she has only himself or herself. Ahead of him lies the forest, which appears dark and dangerous; inevitably attractive. He does not know what adventures await him; he does not have a path mapped out. Perhaps he senses that he is not choosing the easy option. He doesn't know how many times he will suffer, feel happy, rescue, be rescued . . . . When the journey comes to an end, he or she will not be the same, he or she will have been transformed, through a constant process of deconstruction and construction.

Becoming a psychoanalyst nowadays is a bit like going against the current. In times in which immediacy prevails, we choose a training of many years, we propose to patients effective but complex solutions to their suffering. Along the way, and in parallel, we go through our didactic analysis, supervisions, seminars; we also form families, we go through difficult economic and/or affective moments, good, bad, light, etc. It is worthwhile then to ask ourselves: Why do we support with passion what we have chosen? A valid question, although its answer varies infinite times.

## Dear Institute

I have been on this path since long before I met you. I was 10 years old, my mother took me to my first consultation with an analyst. After a few interviews that initiated what later became my first analysis, I thought: "This person waits for me in the evenings, plays with me and then my mother pays her for it. I definitely want to be a psychoanalyst."

Of course, it was not exactly as I had thought at the time. However, I was not so wrong. It is a profession that requires, among other skills, as much playfulness and creativity as possible.

Years later, already graduated as a psychologist, I started my second analysis. My analyst was a didactic analyst at my Institute. But I remember thinking "Psychoanalysis and psychoanalytic training? No way for me!" It was a long time after my analysis that I found myself with the interest and curiosity for this art, discipline or however you want to understand the Psychoanalytic task.

I was lucky. It was not necessary to face the challenge of a change of analyst. Not even the beginning of an analysis. My analysis had already begun. Although it did require some adjustments to become my didactic analysis. I had to change my supervisor, as my previous supervisor although a great psychoanalyst, did not belong to the IPA. It was a painful process. I cannot imagine how difficult it must be when someone has to change analysts. Despite understanding the regulation and criteria, this process has been very difficult for me.

The beginning of the seminars and the first supervision coincided with the moment in life when I had children at a very young age. It required a lot of effort and all the strength of desire. I always remember reading some text by Donald Meltzer in which he mentions the hard work we parents have to do during the period of upbringing.

Little by little I felt that the world was growing, expanding enormously inside me and outside of me.

Theoretical reading has always been pleasurable for me. Along with it, didactic analysis and didactic supervision have been the necessary support to immerse myself in the psychoanalytic experience.

Then, came the experiences shared with my training colleagues and a bond of trust and intimacy began to be woven. We set up what was the "Claustro" (organization of candidates of my Institute) of my cohort at that time and we multiplied the activities in which we shared thoughts and clinical practice within APdeBA. Peer-to-peer meetings became indispensable. We had the support and encouragement of the teaching and didactic analysts.

Most of the time I had to go to APdeBA in the mornings and I remember the brightness, the sun coming in warmly through the windows and the mate (typical infusion in Buenos Aires) and coffee that circulated and brought us together as if it were the fire of the adolescent summer camps. Of course, there were differences, passionate discussions too. Stefano Bolognini (Bolognini, 2014) wrote that it is together with peers that one becomes aware of one's own limitations. I felt that we inhabited the space.

Among the tasks that were available in the "Claustro" of analysts in training, I chose to take care of those that referred to inter-institutional relations. This gave me a great opportunity to meet the analysts in training from other Argentinean analysts in training organizations (Claustros).

At that time, the IPA Congress was held in Buenos Aires. Most of us were going to participate because the conditions were very accessible. Actually, most of us did.

It was around that time that I discovered that in the backyard of APdeBA, perhaps behind the lemon tree that, it is said, was planted by Janine Puget's grandparents by chance, there seems to be a secret window. When you manage to open it, a huge world unfolds. There they were coming to life, making recognizable faces of the acronyms that had been a kind of unknown language. I am referring to the candidates' organizations of Latin America and the world: OCAL/IPSO. Colleagues were solving similar challenges to ours, in very different cultural contexts and places on the planet. It was, and still is, a pleasure to listen to the music of different accents, different languages. Many of them had more experience than me, others similar.

I realized, with regret, that I was being very lucky because this wonderful door is not known to all the analysts in training at my Institute. I dare say it is not known to all senior analysts either. But by finding it and opening it, in my experience, the learning process is absolutely transformed. It allowed me to find or create aspects of myself that I didn't know existed. Perhaps they didn't exist. The possibility of playing is enhanced. Playing is a serious activity in itself and seems vital during training. It is directly related to the passion necessary to go through the experience. The poet fantasizes, Freud would say in "The literary creator and the fantasizing" (Freud, 1993). We become psychoanalysts.

For his part, Winnicott points out that play and playing are transitional phenomena that form the basis of the general cultural experience (Winnicott, 1971c). However, the capacity to play is a developmental achievement. It is not given from the beginning but must be acquired. In the analytic training this process is not lonely. It is in the space "between" analysts that creativity and production are made possible through encounters and misunderstandings. This learning and this game of rivalries, complicities, pleasure in horizontal relationships, impacted and transformed for me, both the shared environment and the loneliness (no longer so solitary) of the consulting room.

I agree with Stefano Bolognini who warns of the danger of analysts becoming isolated, whatever the professional moment in which we are. Above all, the risk of remaining in an endogamic space, where the exchange with other colleagues from the Institute itself, from other Institutes, from other regions, from other continents, does not take place. Fraternal ties break with the myth of solipsistic conceptualizations.

In this sense, I would like to highlight the importance of the fraternal dimension, the bond with peers that will later favor the process of exogamy.

The fourth leg of the tripod. Here It was, completing the four-legged tripod for my training, which as I write this letter reaches the end of this first stage in my becoming an analyst.

In the middle of this path, we were surprised by the pandemic. I met some of my colleagues who were joining us only virtually. Only now, after two years, I am beginning to meet them in person.

I am grateful to my teachers, supervisors, my analyst and my colleagues inside and outside the Institute, inside and outside my country, inside and outside my region.

Dear Institute, I also have suggestions. Some of them arise from my own experience. Others, from those shared with my colleagues. I could assemble them according to the different aspects of the tripod.

Regarding seminars, I have already mentioned that I really enjoyed the readings and debates. I have felt the freedom to think, to fight with the texts and authors to understand them better. I also enjoyed all the plurality of thought and the tolerance for differences that I have found in each seminar.

My Institute has the specificity of granting the IPA training and the university accreditation. This possibility has advantages and disadvantages.

From my point of view, the coexistence of psychoanalytic transmission and university teaching implies a conflict. I do not have an answer for it. Just an observation, perhaps a warning to be alert and preserve the singular spirit that our training implies.

I understand that including Psychoanalysis in the University could be very valuable. However, sometimes I have felt that the psychoanalytic perspective was lost among the university demands. For example, in my opinion the times and processes required for psychoanalytic training do not always coincide with those of university education.

Regarding didactic analysis and supervision, I have not had to make a change of analyst. I have had to change supervisors since my previous supervisor, despite being a great psychoanalyst, did not belong to IPA. This experience made me think about the difficulty of changing analyst when necessary. At APdeBA it is possible to choose an analyst or supervisor from any IPA Institute. I know that not all Institutes allow it. I think it is a strength of APdeBA that must be preserved because it favors the openness and flexibility typical of psychoanalytic thought. I am glad that in my Institute it is this way.

Finally, talking about the fourth leg of the tripod, I consider institutional participation as important as the ties among peers. At this point, my experience is that the Institute fully supports these ties, and it is possible to move freely to present proposals and projects. They are always well received. However, there is no systematized proposal by the Institute that promotes this possibility. Rather, it depends on the curiosity or concern of each analyst in training. Many times, it is in each didactic analysis where the candidate can work this aspect, but there are also many didactic analyses that do not consider it an interest to work in this space.

The same happens in relation to the motivation to exchanges with other Institutes from other countries and regions. Therefore, it is supported and well received, but I have not found a systematization to reach this possibility.

Consequently, for many analysts in training, training happens endogamously with the loss of wealth that this implies.

I hope these observations can be a contribution to my Institute. In any case, my personal experience and my balance about my Institute has been even better than my expectations, precisely because it has had all these nuances that allow me to keep my thoughts moving.

I would choose my Institute again and again.

I am not the same person who entered APdeBA for the first time and enjoyed that sun, that pleasant luminosity. However, I enter again enriched and I enjoy again that sun, that brightness, all that I have received, my usual colleagues, the colleagues that are joining and the possibility of thinking the world in a psychoanalytical key.

I would like to say goodbye for now, dear Institute, by sharing a little piece of the story of "Alice in Wonderland" (Carrol, 2000). Far from boring you with explanations about why it reminds me of my process during my training, I have simply decided to let you enjoy Lewis Carroll's paragraph as a gift: "May I know who you are," asked the Caterpillar, . . . Alice answered, somewhat intimidated:

- The truth, madam, is that at the moment I am not quite sure who I am. The fact is that I know very well who I was this morning, when I woke up, but since then I must have undergone several transformations.

- "What are you trying to tell me?"—said the Caterpillar sternly, "Please explain!"
- "That's just the point!"—exclaimed Alice. "I can't explain myself because I'm not me, do you realize that?"
- "Well, no, I don't," said the Caterpillar.
- "I'm sorry I can't explain it to you more clearly," said Alice in a very polite tone, "because, to begin with, I don't understand it myself . . . You understand that changing size so many times in a single day is not easy to understand!"
- "Yes, it is easy," replied the Caterpillar.
- "Well, you haven't gone through it yet," said Alice, **"but the day will come when you will become a chrysalis and then a butterfly, and then we'll see how you feel!"**

— Marìa Florencia Biotti

# 26 A letter to Asociación Psicoanalítica de Madrid, Spain (1981)

*Cecilia Caruana*

*The Asociación Psicoanalítica de Madrid (APM) was recognized as a component society of the IPA in 1981. Its training is largely based on the French model, but it also takes aspects of the Uruguayan model and the Eitingon model. The future candidate will be eligible to join the Training Institute, through three personal interviews after a minimum of three years in analysis with a training psychoanalyst.*

*Once in the Institute, you will have to pass four compulsory seminars on Freud, one on Psychoanalytic Technique and one on Psychopathology, in addition to four free-choice seminars. At the same time, you can start with the official supervisions. While within training, an ongoing supervision is considered a mainstay, official supervisions are part of the work to be submitted on the way to becoming an associate member. In the APM, two supervisions of two years each are mandatory, each one with a patient on a couch at a minimum frequency of three sessions per week. If you pass the Official Supervisions together with the seminars and with a deliberation of the Teaching Commission, this will grant them the End of Training. At this point the candidate will be able to write and present a paper that will open the door to become an Associate Member (also called a 'graduate analyst' elsewhere).*

—

My dear institute,

It has been 12 years since I started my training at the institute of the Asociación Psicoanalítica de Madrid (APM), and at this moment, from the perspective I have from here, I can see a prolongation of all those initial feelings, but also their transformations brought about by the passing of the years and the different experiences that come with belonging and being linked to this training.

At that time, after five years of analysis and the entrance interviews, one day I finally picked up the letter from the mailbox with all the joy in the world contained in an envelope.

DOI: 10.4324/9781003465409-26

For me, the entrance to the institute was a milestone, almost like the passage of an initiation rite. I was very invested in the access to this formation, I wanted it very much. I wonder if that confirmation brought with it another confirmation: that of being able to distance myself from certain evil forces that I feared might dwell within me. In a certain sense, this entrance was a relief.

In my case, a fuzzy desire to be a psychoanalyst goes back to childhood. Mary Poppins with her restorative magic, her benevolent presence in the lives of others. Fixing family problems and disappearing without leaving any trace but the memory. My analyst, when I told him all this, went for the phallic shape of the umbrella. I was put off by his prosaic view of my daydreams, but it is also true that we did not stop talking to each other because of it.

My fears, madness and childish longings were combined with a home-grown curiosity about dreaming—that phenomenon that makes us equal, for which one does not have to pay, nor does it depend on how happy one is. Dreams will always be there for those who want to remember them. They belong to the children and to the elders.

Today I think that these were the three reasons that led me to the training institute.

Going back to the moment when I received the letter, I had to sit down to read it calmly because I was so excited that I was afraid of losing my balance. Today it makes me laugh to see myself like this, so crazy with desire. So many desires in my body and idealizations in my head.

## How to keep the illusion after the fall, my first contacts

Dear institute, today I think that for our training analysts it should not always be easy to accept these states of idealization with which we candidates land, especially when these idealizations are loaded with feelings of omnipotence that we will have to help channel towards other destinies.

If our destiny is to be frustrated, in my case it was to crash when I opened Mary Poppins' umbrella. However, after the initial crash and subsequent falls, I was able to listen to the words of my analyst; and that message, which at the time I undoubtedly experienced as a hindrance, I came to understand that it could have a practical character between the profession and my own future.

Once inside the training, the first disappointment had to do with the direct access to the training analysts. In my mind, the figure of an eternally elderly psychoanalyst, with full mental faculties, sober in dress, restrained in speech, critical but open to the new, was drawn in my mind. In the case of the women analysts, they had to dress elegantly, have children with liberal professions, be orderly in taking patient notes, well-read and financially unconcerned.

Seeing them so closely, side by side in the seminars, chatting with them after class and even going out to dinner, allowed me to discover with a mixture of horror and delight their weaknesses of character, their imperfections in lecturing, hesitations in the face of intelligent/impertinent questions from some colleagues, excessive allusions to their own patients, clinical examples that were repeated . . . in short, what for me at that time were flaws incompatible with psychoanalytic purity.

In that sense, I believe that the first years of my training were the time in which I was hardest on my own analyst and on the institution. Only the passage of time has been able to heal me, with my repeated falls and clumsiness, which the patients have surely forgiven me more times than I would have forgiven them.

It is true that the critical spirit remains, but fortunately there has been a shift towards a different place, related more to the commitment to the (psychoanalytic) cause than to other intellectual aspects or forms. On the other hand, I constantly think about the idea of an impossible job, a question that relaxes rather than frustrates me today.

Dear institute, from where I am now, I believe that training analysts who give seminars should be required to have a good preparation and a willing attitude towards the transmission of knowledge. In this sense, if in the session the focus should be placed on emotion, in the seminars it should be placed on the texts or the subject matter. Of course, this is not rigid and there must be a permeability to infinite situations and sharing of personal experiences, but we should not lose sight of what we are here for.

The optional seminars were in general more rewarding than the obligatory ones, I approached theoretical content that I desired and related with and I approached the thought of psychoanalysts that called my attention.

I cannot separate the seminars from the candidates with whom I shared the training.

## Seminars, friends and wine

Landing in the training entailed some movements at an internal level that were very positive to deal with in personal analysis, however my passage through the obligatory seminars—*Los Freud*—would not have been the same without those times of elaboration and enjoyment with my fellow candidates. I was fortunate to be in a small class that enjoyed talking and staying up late in the nightlife of Madrid.

There was something delirious in those ethylic prolongations.

Now I remember many times telling each other, with details, how the admission interviews had been, with whom we had been assigned, hilarious anecdotes that we repeated when some stranger joined us. Almost like a euphoric celebration for having arrived, but also in an attempt to assimilate that rare experience of admission interviews and the exciting prospect of becoming a psychoanalyst.

Later, I got to know other colleagues in different forums, in optional seminars and finally through IPSO and congresses outside Spain I got in touch with candidates who opened my mind.

The trips outside Spain had the effect of parents who send their children to learn about other realities, knowing that they will question them. That is why I now feel so grateful to belong to an institution like the APM, which may have its problems and shortcomings, but it opens the doors of the world to us.

Undoubtedly, my Cross Regional Study Group (with colleagues from Canada, Mexico and Brazil) with whom we meet once a month, is one of the most interesting experiences and one that has surprised me the most because of how well it has worked. We have been working online for seven years and each time—as a result of getting to know each other better—the contributions are richer, and a very fruitful work environment has been generated.

Studying groups abroad, working parties of several days in a row with totally unknown candidates, are situations that are impossible to develop if you do not belong to an IPA institute. Enrichment through contact with other people is an incentive and a further pillar on this path.

In my peer group, those who started the training at the same time, and passed through the seminars together, we were very different from each other, and we have taken different paths. This was a group passionate about psychoanalysis, and yet none of us are members. This should give us food for thought.

## Commitment to the Institute

Dear Institute, the passage through the training is becoming a too long stop for many candidates of the APM; a minority are those who pass to member before the ten years, for the rest the average is quite a bit higher, and lucky if you finally present the work to be a member as the fate of many candidates is to eternize training. The APM currently has 180 candidates and only 112 members![1]

The atmosphere can be depressing. I do not know if it is the cause or the consequence, but it contributes to the feeling of a viscous environment in which it would be difficult to move.

In my case, this feeling came to me years after I started training. The stagnation that I perceived in relationships with other older members seemed organic when, to give an example, they always sat in the front rows and the candidates in the back. Where there was an atmosphere at meetings and clinical sessions of grating solemnity until there was a tension in the air. In some ways, It has felt like an order where nothing changes, yet it is necessary to keep moving, because time has passed and you have to be able to occupy other places.

In this journey as a candidate, I have gradually realized something that has given me life: that there are many roles within the institute, and that undoubtedly, the role of the candidate representative is a privileged one.

Like everything in life, things are one way when you imagine them, but executing them is another matter. I was a representative for two separate periods in time, and always on a team. While in the first period I had only been in my training for three years, in the second I had already experienced things outside Spain, and I needed to share them to my colleagues in order to make the experience of being a candidate more vibrant.

Both periods were interesting—working together and learning from other members of other committees to carry out certain projects. These are experiences that strengthen the personality and give confidence.

The organization of congresses, working groups, study days, exchanges with other institutes, etc., are activities that can bring you closer to the institution and its dynamics and that can generate a very different type of gratification to those experienced in the relationship with a patient, so they are activities that work well combined.

### Official supervisions/Control Cases

Now I realize that if analysis is the space with the greatest capacity to generate changes both in life in general and in the relationship with patients, supervision occupies second place in terms of the possibility of change in thinking and deepening psychoanalytic technique.

The obligation to remain working weekly for two years with a supervisor allows for the development of a work that invites deepening and knowledge of a different way of being treated (in all meanings). In a way, the supervisee is the depositary of a way of working. The supervisee recognizes in the relationship with his supervisor the analyst in front of him, and it is difficult when you are in front of a supervisor whom you admire not to wonder what would have become of you if he had been your analyst.

Dealing with a supervisor represents a step further away from analysis, yet it also generates anxiogenic levels in the supervisee who is able to realize when things are not going well with a patient he himself is involved with. It is in the supervisor's hands to be able to welcome them and give an answer back to his supervisee. For me it has been very interesting to see the different ways of approaching these more personal issues from the supervisory point of view.

From the relationships with my supervisors, themes such as humanity in dealing with a patient, commitment, involvement with psychoanalysis versus psychotherapy, the object of work in a session with a patient—it is as if this step of distance from my own analysis has allowed me to see other things that I could not think about during my own analysis. The supervisions allow me to think about things that have been experienced during the analysis.

The two official supervisions I have done have had a revolutionary effect on the way I work. The first one opened my mind a lot, got me out of the fight with my analyst, helped me to rebel again against what I felt was biased and unfair. And at the same time, that same supervision helped me to see that I had to go back to my analyst and be able to confront what I was so angry about. It was a supervision marked by intensity, in which at times the neurotic presence of the supervisee picked up a lot of speed.

The second supervision was much longer and more calm, and marked by a constant feeling of learning and frustration. During many sessions I felt unable to listen to myself with the patient, blocked and without any creative capacity,

I longed for the arrival of the next supervision so that the supervisor would tell me what he saw in the session. It was only when I was finished with the supervision that I was able to benefit, along with my other patients, from all that I had learned.

For me, supervisions can be very desirable but at the same time, very persecutory spaces. The possibility of encountering new ways of looking at the patient that point to deep aspects of the mental functioning of the relationship is not something that is so easy to incorporate.

### . . . Last but not least

Like so many adolescents who come for consultation and who show doubts about their professional choices, one accompanies them momentarily to their own vital bifurcations and to these transcendental decisions. It is true, life can be lived in many different ways and each time I think it is a matter of striking a balance between the choices we have made and the ability to adapt to a reality we did not count on when we made our decision.

My psychoanalytic training is the mark of a way of life, of a commitment that has a changing form but that is Psychoanalysis. I can affirm that the IPA (International Psychoanalytic Association) institutes are the ones that provide the best structured training, that allow the desire to be a psychoanalyst to be better rooted in a profession of flesh and blood.

For the moment, and I live it as a triumph of my institute, the desire to be a member is still in me. And I hope that this desire will be with me for the rest of my life.

Sincerely yours,

Cecilia Caruana

### Note

1  Term at APM for someone who has completed training and is a graduate analyst.

# 27 A letter to the Psychoanalytic Institute of Northern California, San Francisco, USA (1989)

*Nicolle Zapien*

*The Psychoanalytic Institute of Northern California (PINC), located in San Francisco (California, USA), is a pluralistic institute that teaches a range of psychoanalytic theories including group process and the social and contextual dimensions of psychoanalysis. Our founders were among those who fought for inclusion of non-medically trained professionals in the IPA 40 years ago. Many of our candidates and senior analysts write and present their work at conferences nationally and internationally, in professional journals, and books. PINC uses the Eitingon Model of training including a training analysis, which operates like a personal analysis, weekly supervision for each of our training cases, and four years of seminars concurrently. In addition, PINC invites candidate participation in some of the governing committees of the institute including its board of directors. Dr. Zapien is a member of the Visiting Scholar Committee and the Ethics Committee at PINC. There is more than one training institute in the San Francisco Bay Area and we often voluntarily attend additional seminars, case conferences, and presentations at our local sister institutes. Dr. Zapien founded The Center for Psychoanalysis and Technology in 2022 which produces Technology and the Mind, a podcast dedicated to applying psychoanalytic theory to consumer technology use cases.*

---

Dear Institute,

I wish to share with you my thoughts inspired by Fred Busch's edited volume, *Dear Candidate: Analysts from Around the World Offer Personal Reflections on Psychoanalytic Training, Education and the Profession* (Busch, 2020). In this text the analyst authors each discussed his or her experience as a candidate including what he or she has learned through years (sometimes many decades) of psychoanalytic practice that may be useful to candidates. As I embark upon my fourth year of training, close to its end but still not finished, it is clear that I have learned much in what now feels like a short time. I have transformed substantively in ways I did not expect. But there is also not yet sufficient *Nachträglichkeit*[1] to reflect on and integrate the experience of

DOI: 10.4324/9781003465409-27

being a candidate in training, nor to grasp the fullness of the experience of my own training analysis as it too is still in progress, a point that many of the analyst authors in Busch's text mentioned. Furthermore, I have yet to become a training analyst or to take up the roles of teaching, supervising, and some of the more influential administrative committee positions within my institute. What follows therefore may read like the naïve passionate demands of an adolescent who has a somewhat uninformed critique veiled as idealism to share with the elders. I imagine that in several years after I graduate from training, complete my analysis and am on my way to becoming a training analyst myself, if I were to embark upon writing a similar *Dear Institute* letter at that time, I might write something quite different than what follows.

My letter begins, dear Institute, with a description of what I think are the most influential relationships I have had with people and particular administrative processes or groups of people who serve administrative functions at PINC, each of which are associated with their attendant transferences and dynamics. One such important relationship is the relationship I had to PINC prior to applying to train. This includes all aspects of marketing, public relations, community events, word of mouth reports, and admissions processes. These are, in my opinion, significantly important in that these collectively act as gatekeeping functions to the profession and also act to provide the public with perceptions about psychoanalysis as a profession even if this is not consciously intended. How the interactions with these functions and people went when I was talking to colleagues, searching the website for information, receiving newsletters, attending community member events, engaging with a free mentor that is provided prior to applying, and finally applying, were largely positive. Having said that, because my career prior to becoming a psychotherapist involved consulting to technology companies and nonprofits about marketing strategy and website usability, I was able to consider the first touch points with PINC (e.g., the website, events, admissions process) as part of a system that functions in a less than smooth, coordinated and transparent way. Organizations that are run by committees and volunteers often do not run smoothly or transparently, for very good human reasons, and they similarly do not typically spend as much time, energy, and money as it takes to develop and maintain well-designed strategic mentoring, marketing, public relations, and optimized website programs. This previous knowledge and experience, as well as the fact that I am a white, middle class, middle aged, heterosexual, cis-gendered person and as such do not often face discrimination, allowed me to easily believe that I might be accepted to train at PINC and that PINC might be a great institute, despite any navigation challenges I may have had so far. I often wonder if there are many qualified and interested potential applicants or community members seeking an analyst who are dissuaded from engaging more deeply with us, either because they perceive discriminating barriers through these initial touchpoints, or they perceive that the institute or the profession is not organized. This is important, I think, because younger generations tend to have higher standards for website designs and functionality and also tend to demand clear and transparent communication due to their being steeped in technology and customer relational management systems in ways that older generations are not. Our website, sorry to say, is less than ideal in terms of content and functionality and I know that the institute is well aware of this fact. I can only hope that we are able to make a solid investment in the future in redesigning our website and outreach efforts as part of a strong coordinated marketing strategy of the profession and of our institute in particular. We should at least aim to remove any informational and navigational barriers to all constituents seeking to engage with us.

Once I applied, the most important and influential relationship I have with anyone within the institute is with my personal training analyst (of course), and likely my feelings about this relationship, which are largely infused with strong feelings of gratitude at the current moment, have the most influence on how I feel about the institute as a whole. But I want to also challenge myself, dear Institute, to think beyond the particulars of this relationship to consider the institute as a whole, as Busch's (2020) book has done for us. This allows me to be more private and protective of my relationship with my personal training analyst, and at the same time to acknowledge the contributions that others at the institute have made to my training experience, the experience of my colleagues, and those who come after us. It also helps me to consider the ways that we, as candidates, may impact how the institute functions.

My experience, once accepted to train, has also been largely positive with the exception of the occasional seminar faculty who I perceive to be either underprepared, lacking rigorous thinking or openness to critical thinking, or simply unskilled at the art of teaching. There have also been particular supervisors/consultants who are in my opinion, too rigid or authoritative for my tastes. My general message to those who teach or offer supervision and consultation is this—**we need you to push yourselves, to think more about what you teach or offer us.** What are the holes in the theories you present? What are the controversial discussions that are yet to be resolved in the field that are relevant to what you share? How do your ideas apply (or not) to different contexts or particular issues that are in the social surround? How can you manage any anxieties or narcissism you may have about teaching or supervision/consultation even more than you already do, so that we might resist what you have to offer less, or so that we might be in a truly creative and rigorous dialogue with you? In short, we need you to be open and flexible so that you can help us to understand the current debates and issues quickly, so that we might continue to develop the field to address urgent needs from our patients and our communities. We also need you to trust our developing psychoanalytic thinking even as you challenge us so that we have solid analytic identities in the end.

I want to briefly discuss the organizational and administrative details of the institute. At PINC, many administrative functions are handled by volunteers and most tasks are done by committees and are thus subject to group dynamics. Candidates participate in some of these activities and from what I can tell there is a real commitment to developing a community with functioning work groups, and to processing what occurs in these groups with a psychoanalytic sensibility. I appreciate the hours spent volunteering to run the institute and I participate in two committees myself as a candidate. I would say, however, that these committees are not always run efficiently and **sometimes the work groups spend more time thinking analytically about the tasks at hand than doing the tasks themselves.** I recognize this may be adolescent whining and that there may be more wisdom in the group process than I can appreciate from where I sit currently in my training, but sometimes I would very much like to have efficiency and action take precedent when we have programs to plan or decisions to make. I often wonder what might be possible if we were more active and efficient in terms of creative projects and outreach—I would find it so enlivening to accomplish more together, by doing!

There have been some difficult discussions between candidates, potential candidates and training analysts at my institute (for example, about perceived elitism in psychoanalysis and the need to be more inclusive of BIPOC[2] people, immigrants, and others.) There is an emphasis currently at my institute in discussing the costs of training and other perceived barriers to inclusivity, which are likely rooted in the vast disparities in wealth in the San Francisco Bay Area, and this includes ongoing consideration of how to make treatment more available to a broader range of patients. These dialogues have not been easy. I have appreciated the numerous hours that many training analysts and candidates have volunteered to participate in these important dialogues, their steady long-term commitment to participation in institutional life, and that many have lowered their fees to make room for inclusivity of a more socioeconomically diverse training group. These gestures have been meaningful and concretely helpful to many and are consistent with some of the larger concerns in our society. It makes me very sad, however, to hear that some training analysts avoid these dialogues because they wish to protect psychoanalysis as a rigorous discipline and do not feel that there is room for their concerns in such dialogues. It produces in us the sense of an Oedipal victory that is problematic and, for me, strong feelings of loss as their wisdom may be swept to the side by urgent battle calls for change. We need everyone's voices and participation, and we *do* need to protect what is essential in psychoanalysis, even as we must make changes to address charges of elitism and exclusivity. **Dear Institute—please do not avoid participating fully in the dialogues that are difficult even if you feel we are too angry, naïve, or insistent.** *We need your steadiness, patience, and wisdom,* if we are to move through these difficult conversations and develop together for the future. I imagine there are likely very different contexts where others train, however, both the institutional context and the social surround is relevant for what candidates may want to communicate or need from their institutes.

From my perspective, situated as it is, I have just a few overarching sentiments to communicate, dear Institute. From what I can tell of my fellow candidates and myself, we have many demands and needs as we train in these historical times. We need all the usual things that a personal training analysis (hopefully) provides. We need support for transforming and working through our pre-Oedipal, Oedipal, and Post-Oedipal conflicts. We need you to help us to learn for ourselves (by experiencing with you) the deepening of a treatment, and the seeing it through to completion. We need you to be with us intimately and authentically and with appropriate analytic distance and integrity, so that we can integrate your presence as we sit with our patients. We need to have you surprise us, challenge us, have courage in your interpretations, and deep conviction in the field, the frame, and its techniques. But we also need some specific things from our analysts, supervisors, and seminar faculty, as well as from the institute, things that belong to these historical times, and are new and extra. We need you to be sensitive to the future needs we may have, needs that we have as we find ourselves smack in the middle of a massive cultural transformation. We need you to offer us a psychoanalysis that is just as sturdy as it is flexible, so that it can be adapted with care for the future, in line with the ethics of those times. We need you to question us—and yourselves—intently about a great number of assumptions, and to push our theories, even the ones you love, hard so that we are prepared. We need to be prepared, I think, for doing psychoanalysis during wars we cannot yet imagine, economic crises that may be worse than ever before, overpopulation and intense competition for resources, climate crises, pandemics, and civil unrest. All of these will likely be made more complicated through the use of consumer technologies which seem to expedite and magnify everything including misinformation and polarization. Furthermore, technology may produce a grand turning away from the other and relationships in so many ways, toward screens that I imagine will create additional problems even as they purport to solve some of them. Technological advancements may threaten our capacity for negative capability, attention, empathy, creativity, and a familiarity with the interiority of the self that psychoanalysis is based on. We cannot afford to sit on the sidelines and think only about tele-analysis vs. in person analysis when it comes to technology (although we must also take this question up fully); we must also take up and theorize the issues of how we experience the self and relationships altogether in technologically mediated ways outside our consulting rooms too.

Dear Institute, I have already asked for so much even as you give so much. We are a demanding generation and one that votes on social media or with our feet (*a la* 'cancel culture'). If we are anything like higher education research suggests, I think the generations of candidates to come will be even more demanding (Chessman & Wayt, 2016; St. Amour, 2020; Woodall et al., 2012). For example, at my institute candidates often question the requirements and the costs of training, and we are often critical of certain theories as outdated, elitist, racist, sexist, or pathologizing. We may request to have extensions to file reports or to change advisors or supervisors or wish to have seminars in person or online or at different times to meet our particular wishes and needs.

I hear from older, more seasoned analysts, that this was not the case in their training. We don't raise these issues because we want to be insolent or entitled, or because we don't value what you have to offer, or because we want to have a less rigorous training, or to bypass our narcissism—in fact *we make these demands because we need all the support we can get*. We simply cannot have an inclusive and robust psychoanalysis that reflects the concerns of the current economic and social context if we do not address some of these structural issues.

Despite any quips that we as candidates make that are hurtful or seem disrespectful or adolescent, there is deep gratitude and reverence for your patience and wisdom. Your conviction in psychoanalysis, and your generosity is apparent and underscores your love for psychoanalysis and your belief in its future—in us. Please continue to offer this. Psychoanalysis is transmitted in this way. In my case, I have more gratitude for my training than I can articulate. I went into this training thinking I wanted to deepen my clinical work, recognizing that analysts I knew thought in ways about clinical work that I admired. I thought I would learn theory and technique and would develop a stronger group of peers with whom to consult. Those are all pieces of what training has been to me, but they have not been the heart of it. To truly listen with evenly hovering attention, to welcome the fullness of our experiences, to survive as an object, and to be willing to go in your mind and heart as you accompany us in ours—that has been the center of it all. This is perhaps what is most important, and exactly what we need from you, regardless of what we demand. If I am lucky, one day I will be an active training analyst member of my institute, and with my colleagues we will welcome a new generation of candidates who will challenge us and demand that we push our ideas further. I hope that they will be just as grateful for what we have to offer.

— Nicolle Zapien

## Notes

1 Freud used the German word *Nachträglichkeit*, meaning the state or condition of being after the event or having hindsight. https://www.oxfordreference.com
2 Black, Indigenous, and People of Color.

# 28 A letter to Sociedade Portuguesa Psicanálise, Portugal (1999)

*Liliana Correia de Castro*

*Activities linked to Psychoanalysis in Porto took place in the early 1970s, through the initiatives of Jaime Milheiro, then an Associate Member of the Sociedade Portuguesa de Psicanálise. At this time, accredited psychoanalysts visited Porto, where, in the form of clinical meetings, seminars or conferences, Francisco Alvim, João dos Santos, Eduardo Cortesão, Pedro Luzes, José Flores, Coimbra de Matos, Pierre Luquet and others, lengthened paths and perspectives.*

*In 1980, the "Group of Psychoanalytic Studies of Porto and Coimbra", later known as the "Group of the North", formed by Jaime Milheiro, Carlos Amaral Dias, Eurico Figueiredo and Celeste Malpique, formed the basis for the creation of the future IFTP.*

*From 1982 to 1988 this group organized four "Northern Psychoanalysis Meetings", under the themes "Identification and Identity", "Hysteria from Dora", "Obsession, Symptom and Culpability" and "Depression, Depressions". By this time, the training process in Psychoanalysis was centralized in Lisbon, which did not prevent activities of a clinical and scientific nature from advancing in the North, within an active spirit that disseminated it in the most varied contexts. The successive passage to Teaching Members of the SPP of the elements of the group, little by little made training possible in this region.*

*In 1997, the members of the city's SPP (members, associates and candidates), in a formal meeting, elected an "Organizing Committee of the Institute of Psychoanalysis of Porto", composed of Jaime Milheiro, Celeste Malpique, Fátima Cabral, José Ferronha and Rui Coelho, which were mandated to obtain the administrative, scientific, physical space and other requirements necessary for its installation and operation. The Porto Institute for Psychoanalytic Training and Therapy was formally opened in 1999, with the aim, according to its Statutes, "to promote training and therapy in Psychoanalysis" and "extending its action to the entire northern region of the country".*

DOI: 10.4324/9781003465409-28

*IFTP (Instituto de Formação e Terapêutica Psicanalítica do Porto)/SPP (Sociedade Portuguesa de Psicanálise) training requirements are:*

- *The completion of your own training analysis.*
- *Completing three years of didactics/lectures (one day per week) plus a fourth year with Clinical Seminars, Seminars on Ethics and Seminars on the work of Bion and Klein.*
- *Following two cases of analysis under supervision ('control cases') with a duration of at least three years each; the supervision frequency should be weekly and the training sessions three times a week.*
- *To present a written report ("Memory") of one of the control cases to the National Society Education Committee (Portuguese Society of Psychoanalysis), which has also to be orally presented and discussed with this Committee.*

—

Dear Institute,

I know our relation just started three years ago, but for me these were extremely rich, intense and incredibly transformative years. My desire to be part of this relation started five years before and my relation to psychoanalysis 12 years ago. I realize this path will continue for many years and I hope that we will have a relation for life and that we can learn, grow and also enjoy together.

I will share with you what led me to psychoanalytic training. My first contact with psychoanalysis occurred during my psychiatric residence during the stage in a psychoanalytic oriented Day Hospital. Previously I have been part of a therapeutic psychotherapeutic group and also of analytical oriented art-therapy and understood I would benefit from an individual and deeper analytical experience. So, I have decided to start my first personal analysis while I continued my residency in Psychiatry. My personal analysis was a life changing experience and deeply helped me both in my personal development as well in my professional life as a psychiatrist and as a therapist. Once I had the luck to contact with psychoanalysis in my life, it became since then part of my life. I started and completed a post-graduation course in psychoanalytic psychotherapy that helped me to consolidate the conviction and desire to become a psychoanalyst. I started to attend more frequently psychoanalytic events and applied to psychoanalytic education at IFTP/SPP (Institute of Oporto/Portuguese Society of Psychoanalysis). After entering as a candidate member at my Institute, I decided to start a second personal analysis while I attended the didactic seminars (theoretical training) and received weekly supervision of my first control case. This decision to do a second analysis during psychoanalytic training turned out to be a fundamental decision and turning point in my analytic education, allowing me to deepen my analytic journey and process. This was revealed to be of much importance and helped me to more deeply elaborate and integrate several aspects of my personal and institutional life and of my personality. As soon as I started my training, I was also lucky enough to contact with IPSO, which allowed an international immersion in psychoanalysis and a closer contact to IPA. Also integrating the IPSO Executive Committee helped me to deepen my experience in group dynamics and work with several challenging moments of institutional functioning and unexpected challenges.

I have also to confess that you, as my chosen group/Institute, were not my only love. During this journey I was also part of and contacted different groups inside and outside my home Institute or Psychoanalyses that were embedded and integrated in my professional and personal/familiar life and routine: my psychoanalytic training group cohort at my Institute (that was quite small and very friendly), study and seminar groups of my Society, the group of IPSO candidates, the group of the IPSO Executive Committee, the group of psychiatry residents and psychiatrists in my Hospital, the group of friends of a poetry writing group, the relation with my analysts and with my supervisor and of course with my friends and family. Marrying, having two kids and three nephews along this journey made everything even more full and intense and let you certainly to a second plan for some moments. It is incredible the amount of effort, dedication and enthusiasm mixed with periods of tiredness, frustration and doubt that being an analyst in training encompasses. As Freud said, psychoanalysis can be an "impossible" profession. It is also incredible how with the passing of time all these different areas of my life start to get closer and united as the construction of an (analytical) puzzle/frame.

This dimension of joy and playfulness while learning (and living) was sometimes easier for me to find among peers, friends and family and that is something I believe we can improve together and not deprive you from this pleasure. Some formality and distant position on your part led sometimes to a more serious hierarchic relation. Intimacy requires more presence and more dialogue, and I believe candidates are open to that. Candidates learn a lot, flourish and grow (or not) inside the Institutes but I believe this to be mutual: institutes can transform and evolve with their analysts in training. This leads us to a reflection on infantilization versus autonomy and on isolation versus integration. This is a risk to take into account by Institutes and something to be vigilant and care for. I would also privilege in person dialogue to online questionnaires when you want to know more about my opinion, ideas or feeling but I know a certain pandemic virus didn´t make our relational life easy.

That being said, I have felt integrated and listened to. There were also long periods of silence and less frequent communication, especially during the pandemic period, but you might have needed your own time to reorganize and adapt. In this period of institutional isolation, international organizations namely the IPA and IPSO and the contact among peers were my best company and provided the time and space we all needed.

Like any relation we have our ups and downs, our idealizations and of course some degree of disappointment or frustration, but fortunately this was the exception and not the rule. I felt generally happy and lucky around you and your psychoanalytic educational program. The quality of the teaching, the friendly educational environment, the organization of the seminars and all the effort to maintain all our activities during the pandemic were extraordinary. Also, the approximation that the online seminars allowed between the Institute of Oporto and of Lisbon were very enriching for me. Now I believe we are finding a common ground of reality and being able to grow, learn, develop and blossom together.

I want also to share with you my best and worse experiences with you.

I must underline again that my best experiences were among peers: analysts in training both from my Institute and Society and also with candidates from around the world. The joyful, relaxing and creative environment and moments between peers were the most rewarding and nurturing moments of my training. Another important experience was the stimulus and guidance from individual senior members of my institute and society, specifically dedicated and supportive of younger generations. This trustful individual attitude of some senior analysts had an important positive impact in different points of my journey. The input, hope, open attitude and mature behavior was both an inspiration and also a trigger for developing, empowerment and nurturing movements and moments. The generosity and open attitude of many senior colleagues have a very profound effect in the younger generation since they are present in a specific phase of analytical education: its beginning.

I also must share with you the most destructive moment I have lived during my training and that refers to an institutional crisis among senior analysts that probably reflects a transgenerational trauma common to many institutes and societies, that carry their own history of division, conflict and rivalry that were activated in some moments of our institutional life. Younger analysts in training inherit this history and live the unconscious dynamics and the destructive forces present. I could feel that both me and other candidates felt confused, sad and also a bit lost in this phase of institutional chaos. To witness these ego fights, divisions, discussions, actings and misunderstandings among senior analysts and the destructive impact it caused in the institutional/group life was very sad and brought mixed feelings of frustration, psychic suffering and disappointment. As a candidate I found myself caught up and immersed in this conflict but was also able to learn about group conflict and dynamic and grow with that. As every crisis there are opportunities for change, renovation and also for reparation and psychic growth. I realized how members in these moments can defend themselves with isolation and avoidance of communication with the younger generations namely candidates in their initial years of training.

Even so, this destructiveness present in some moments of the institutional life had less power than the environment of trust and all the growing and learning moments I could share among younger and older colleagues. I always felt that this transgenerational suffering could be repaired and healed inside the institution and inside the group. Most of the healing and reparation was once again made among peers and also with the wisdom and mature position of many senior colleagues that were courageous enough to communicate more openly with younger members.

In my point of view, one of the areas of improvement in our relation could be to have more time together to communicate, learn and enjoy institutional life. This could be done with creating more moments of learning between younger and older colleagues, a more intense exchange and more inclusion of the younger colleagues in institutional life.

Although I lived the transition movement that the pandemic arose, as my training and analytical process started in presence, transited to online and then back to in person, my personal feeling is that there is nothing that can substitute the wholeness of the presence and the living sharing of life, company, education and treatment in person. I am glad I could be present with my body, soul, mind in a shared place and in a shared time.

Each analytical pathway is a very unique one and my desire is that candidates feel supported and in good company along the way, embraced by joy, pleasure and love more than by solitude, pain and destruction. I wish that their institutes and societies can be felt like a safe and intimate place they can call their home. In the end, we might be lucky enough to be accepted, respected and contribute to a common enriching matrix, in a continuous development and metamorphose of our analytic identity and our own self and life.

Additionally, many creative moments and inspirational experiences were lived with people outside the institute as friends and cultural events. The dialogue between culture and art should not be minimized in analytic training, as psychoanalysis is in permanent dialogue with the world and with human culture. I am interested in the relation of psychoanalysis and poetry. I can see many bridges and similarities between poetry and psychoanalysis: the importance of the words and love for the words, the place of silence and love for the silence, the musicality, the rhythm, the tone, the mystery of the verse as the mystery of the intuition or interpretation, the truth and love for the truth. Emily Dickinson in her poem (Dickinson, 1998) advises us to "tell all the truth but tell it slant", talking about the importance of the use of words and how a very direct and fast truth can make blind the other. As in poetry, what link psychoanalysis to life is love and the relation with the other.

May our love continue to grow in this (analytical) journey.

— Liliana Correia de Castro

# 29 A letter to the Minnesota Psychoanalytic Institute, Minneapolis, USA (1999)

*Nick Flier*

*For the Minnesota Institute in USA, the requirements are:*

- *completing four years of didactics/lectures (one day per week)*
- *three cases under supervision—"control cases"*
- *the completion of your own training analysis*

*A brief history of our society and institute, based on discussion with multiple individuals:*

*Organized psychoanalysis in our region began with the incorporation of the Psychoanalytic Foundation of Minnesota (PFM) in 1970, by a group of psychiatrists from the University of Minnesota, the Chicago Institute, and the Mayo Clinic in Rochester, MN. Over the course of the following three decades, this group sponsored scientific sessions, offered case conferences, literature seminars, and courses for mental health professionals. They also attracted prominent analysts from the Midwest as well as the east and west coast, including the likes of Kohut, Meisner, and Kernberg just to name a few. By the early 1990's, the Psychoanalytic Foundation of Minnesota had its first generation of younger candidates, who were considered "active and enthusiastic members," and had become a part of their study group. By the mid 1990s, the growing organization began to put together a psychoanalytic psychotherapy training program which evolved into an institute and society in 1999. The American Psychoanalytic Association (APsA) decided that they would sponsor a new training facility, building upon what others had created within study groups/psychoanalytic psychotherapy training. The first candidate class helped to plan and launch the Institute. During the early stages, a subcommittee of the CNTF (Committee on New Training Facilities) was assigned to Minnesota. They visited the site on several occasions and helped with the early organizational stage of becoming a provisional Institute. Later, after review, they recommended that the Minnesota Psychoanalytic Institute be allowed to become a free-standing Institute of APsA.*

*The Psychotherapy Center, an offshoot of the Minnesota Psychoanalytic Society, was developed in 2009 with funding from the Society and Institute. The Center recruits and trains psychotherapy fellows to provide services to*

DOI: 10.4324/9781003465409-29

*the community through a low-fee clinic. The Center evolved over time and began recruiting primarily students after becoming an approved internship site for three masters' degree social work students, and three doctoral degree psychology programs. This model has linked graduate students, early career therapists, graduate schools, and the Psychoanalytic Psychotherapy Training Program. Today the Center, the Society, and the Institute operate as separate entities within one organization.*

—

Dear Institute,

I would like to start this letter by mentioning that while I am a psychodynamic psychotherapist, I am not a candidate. I believe there are many others like me, who wish to deepen their analytic knowledge through formal analytic training, and while I cannot speak for them all, I hope to offer a perspective and voice that is shared by many.

Dear Institute, since as early as the second grade, I have loved reading books. Aside from the fantasies and the adventurous experiences that books provide, I believe that I was also drawn to the people within each story. I also believe that I began to develop questions about the mind, body, and the soul before I had the words to describe my experience, because of the books and stories that I loved to read. There is some possibility that I entered our local psycho-analytic society by chance. There is also some probability that I was guided by my unconscious motivation to understand myself, my family, and my patients. The motivation to learn more and to answer questions persists within me. Dear Institute, I have a strong desire to discover and understand the psyche. Perhaps there are several other factors that led me to you, to our society, to this writing project, that only psychoanalysis will reveal. Whatever the case, it is certain that I would not be here without the guidance of a caring mentor and learning from others who are brimming with psychoanalytic wisdom.

The letters written in Fred Bush's *Dear Candidate* provide insight, support, and thoughtfulness of many mentors, as a guide forward in training, and a glimpse behind the curtain of the present state of institutional systems. When considering the history of the behaviors in our institutes it seems that many events are at first intentionally hidden, only to be revealed in time, and that this damages trust. Accounts from analysts who have been through training, and even those considering training, reveal appealing and appalling characteristics that one encounters during analytic training. It is refreshing to see and hear these characteristics out in the open in *Dear Candidate* rather than in whispers of small groups. These letters have helped to tame the romantic idealism I have carried for both analysis and the analyst. Or maybe more accurately, those who assume positions of authority as analysts/teachers/supervisors. (Certainly, my experience on committees has helped with this as well). You have been frank in your acknowledgement of both the shortcomings as well as the rewards one discovers in the pursuit of candidacy, while humbly acknowledging the diversity of perspectives across the world's institutes, societies, and centers. I appreciate the balance in voices and perspectives that have been shared in this compilation. Similarly, I appreciate the way in which you have addressed both the importance of classical theory as the foundation of our field, while acknowledging the evolution of theory to keep up with the changes of our world (if not to ensure the survival of analysis). The value of developing an openness to different schools of psychoanalytic thought, as well as those outside of our institutional "homes," was both reassuring and validating for me. Three pages would not be enough to express my gratitude, particularly because I feel I must also leave room in this letter to share that which raises ambivalence, within me, if not repulsion from deeper participation within the institute.

Dear Institute, I have thoroughly enjoyed and felt energized by your national meetings as an Associate Member. I understand that you are beginning to expand your membership to incorporate a wider lens of experiences, beyond the traditional "analysts-only" assembly. Thank you for evolving in this way. This kind of change must have surely been met with resistance. Change seems to frequently meet resistance. As a chair of our board and member of several ad-hoc committees, I have encountered various gates that have been difficult to pass within APsaA and within my own society and institute. Did you know that I was unable to attend a meeting of leaders at a national meeting? Despite being in a position as president of our local society, I did not qualify to attend this meeting due to my analytic credentials. Stringent rules insisted that one must be a "full member" (an analyst), to attend this leadership meeting. This was confusing for me as I was caught between the belief that "authority" must know best, and a desire to learn and lead. Contrary to what I had heard, I did not find other meetings pretentious, but rather warm and cheerful, though I was perhaps insulated by attending with a friend who is both a candidate and psychiatrist.

Dear Institute, speaking of leadership, I wonder what amount of naivete and/or gravitas it must take to assume a position of leadership in an analytic organization (for me I sheepishly acknowledge both). The paranoia, anger, and confrontation I have experienced in the short time I have spent in a leadership position within my organization has shed light on why it must be so difficult to find volunteers (among the many other more obvious reasons). What is not spoken about is surely felt, and what is spoken about is most definitely felt when it comes to these types of attacks. In defense of those who attack, I acknowledge that it is only natural to be curious about a new person in leadership, though with no trust, and the frequency with which doubt is publicly cast on nearly every decision that is made (decisions that were made with a team) is emotionally draining and is contrary to the spirit I would expect from the analytic community. Dear Institute, you have stated, "You are not the boss of me!" To be sure, this is an accurate statement, and taken out of context could mean many things. But also . . . discouraging.

Dear Institute, the field of psychoanalysis holds so much promise. An approach of depth, breadth, and heart, exploring the workings of the mind, suggesting a path toward ultimate, yet unattainable wisdom. Psychoanalytic centers, societies, and institutes offer a theory (or theories) and a place to better understand the psyche and the unconscious of our patients, to hold and contain our patients, and to develop our own growth and empathy. It seems that institutes vary rather widely with respect to dogma of a dominant theory, and that this lends against an open-minded approach. This was surprising to me. Politics, resistance to change, and outright inappropriate behavior seem present to some degree at each institute. Once this is known, and without proper guidance, psychoanalysis begins to feel shallower rather than deeper.

Dear Institute, to mention now the cost of candidacy, runs the risk of belaboring a point that has been noted in research and amongst most who have considered this educational and developmental path. Though I am aware of some genuine efforts to target this problem, it seems to be another issue that is rarely discussed, at least within the context of finding a solution (see also suppressed). The cost of didactics, supervision, years of analysis, time lost from work and/or family has been (and continues to be) considered the most prohibitive factors in pursuing analytic training. Additionally, the return on investment does not appear to be what it once was. The economics of pursuing analytic training have changed over time, with largely unchanged requisites for candidates, and decreased consumption of analysis by the general public. For me, this leaves personal and professional development as the primary incentive for pursuit of analytic training . . . a noble pursuit and self-fulfilling pursuit, though not necessarily a wise financial choice (pragmatic practitioners may exit here).

A second point that I hope you consider and act upon involves the systemic issues that persist among many institutes. Dear Institute, political infighting and fractions may be a part of our analytic history (see also repetition compulsion—beginning with the founding father and his colleagues), and it may at times lead to growth, though it may also stymie growth, and more importantly has the potential to lead us to our demise. Within my own society and institute there exists an inevitable web of relationships in which teachers/students, supervisors/supervisees, analysts/analysands, psychoanalysts/psychotherapists have roles that overlap, sometimes in many ways. I would guess that our analytic family is not all that different from others in many respects. While this again has its merits, it also leads to much confusion about confidentiality and safety (particularly for the individual in the perceived subversive role in the relationship). As I alluded to earlier, it has been my experience that participation on committees leads to the death of idealism. This is neither all good, nor all bad, though it does give pause to consider the elements of trust and safety that would likely be *essential* to withstand the personal vulnerabilities involved in analytic training.

Lastly, in my humble view Dear Institute, absent of its role in formal analytic training, it seems that session frequency and the duration of treatment can often be determined by the needs of the candidate/supervisor/rigid rules of the training model, as opposed to what is best for the patient. There are some published examples of this, though it seems to be another topic that is not openly discussed (i.e., the fact that it happens, how it happens, and how to prevent this from happening!). The IPA outlines the application of psychoanalysis as "a theory of how the mind works, as a treatment method for psychic problems, as a method of research, and as a way of viewing cultural and social phenomena like literature, art, movies, performances, politics and groups." To me, this application of psychoanalysis can only exist with the "other" (see also "without the baby there is no mother"). This is an idea that I fear may often get lost when efforts are made, and pressure is felt to achieve a particular set of standards for graduation. Are we thinking and acting in good faith for the other? Ultimately, we accept a challenging and fulfilling role (psychodynamic psychotherapists and psychoanalysts alike), to provide a caring service to our patients, which should always supersede our interest in meeting graduate standards.

Perhaps, your response to the thoughts here-in are something along the lines of: "So what? Completion of psychoanalytic training has always been difficult . . . it is not supposed to be easy?" I have indeed heard this feedback vicariously, in some form or another, and I have seen it in writing. If you have read this far, then I believe you have at least a passing interest in hearing from someone like me, and in thinking more deeply about how to recruit (some) analysts in the future. I hope to speak on behalf of those who have strongly considered, or continue to consider analytic training, who also possess a passion for psychoanalytic didactics and have a hunger to learn more about the unconscious in the interest of working more deeply with their patients. Many of us do not possess the keys and privilege to access the gate that will actualize these passions through formal analytic training. These keys are held by those in positions of power. I strongly believe that change starts with you, the analyst, whom we ask for help, and for hope . . . those who have gone before us. Those whom we need as mentors, role models, and supports as we evolve with the changes of the modern-day analyst.

Thank you for your time and consideration.

— Nick Flier

# 30 A letter to the Western Canada Psychoanalytic Society and Institute, Vancouver (2005)[1]

## Michelle van den Engh

The Western Canada Psychoanalytic Society and Institute (WCPSI) is an International Psychoanalytical Association (IPA)-approved institute of the Canadian Psychoanalytic Society (CPS). Founded in 2005 in Vancouver, British Columbia, it was originally named the Vancouver Institute of Psychoanalysis (VIP). With the expansion of psychoanalytic centres to include other Western Canada cities and provinces, it adopted a new name in 2017, the Western Psychoanalytic Society Institute (WPSI). In 2022, the Western Psychoanalytic Society Institute (WPSI) and the Western Branch of the Canadian Psychoanalytic Society (WBCPS) amalgamated to form the Western Canada Psychoanalytic Society and Institute (WCPSI).

Psychoanalytic training at WCPSI includes the three pillars of the Eitingon model as described by the IPA—personal analysis, didactic training and clinical supervision—as well as a fourth component: continuing professional development and participation in societal and institutional life. In addition, WCPSI candidates, now called analysts-in-training (AITs), are required to complete a final graduation paper prior to being recommended for membership in the Canadian Psychoanalytic Society.

The first psychoanalytic training class began in 2005 and the second in 2015. In 2020, the Institute underwent a comprehensive AIT-requested review of its training program, leading to a major overhaul of policies, procedures and organisational structures. WCPSI enrolled its third class of analysts-in-training within this new framework in September 2023.

—

Dear Institute,

I began my psychoanalytic training with a somewhat starry-eyed vision. I imagined robust container/contained psychoanalytic dyads in which raw experience would be gently transformed into meaningful growth. Peers and

DOI: 10.4324/9781003465409-30

colleagues would join harmoniously to delve into the deep secrets of the unconscious and integrate their views. I would learn psychoanalysis—the Rolls Royce treatment of the past, present and future—and pay it forward with a ripple effect. I imagined a linear process of learning psychoanalytic theories, applying them in my clinical practice and then emerging on the other side of training as a full-fledged psychoanalyst. Smooth sailing, so to speak. I was ill-prepared for stormy waters.

I imagined something like this . . .

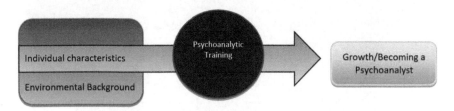

*Figure 30.1* A graphic image depicting how the author imagined psychoanalytic training would be like. Image by the author.

But it was more like this . . .

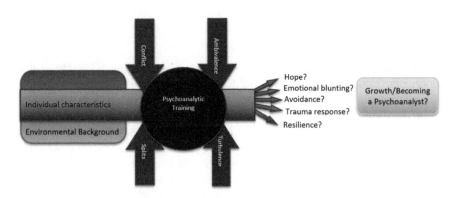

*Figure 30.2* A graphic image depicting how the author found psychoanalytic training to be like.

And sometimes it felt like this . . .

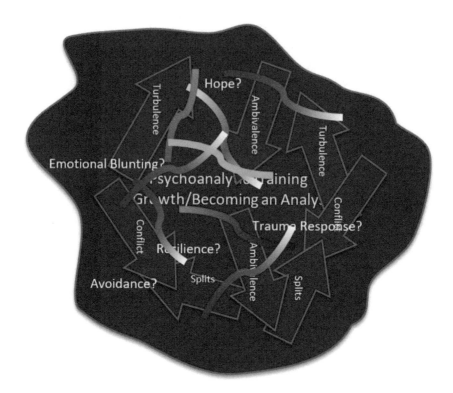

*Figure 30.3* A graphic image depicting how psychoanalytic training sometimes felt
like. Image by the author.

Many authors in the *Dear Candidate* book write candidly about the disillu-
sionments, disappointments and doubts that accompanied their psychoanalytic
education along the way (Busch, 2020). I suspect no Institute is immune. When
turbulence hit our Institute, deep rifts and painful splits were revealed. In the
throes of ambivalence, conflict and turmoil, I felt confused and shaken, as if
I had lost my compass. Amidst the uprisings, I struggled to keep the faith that
times of upheaval would be followed by reconciliation and constructive change.
I felt angry that the peace was being disturbed, and deeply wished that everyone
could just get along. If a group of psychoanalysts couldn't figure this out, who
could? Ideas of psychoanalysis as an invincible haven, a fix-all, crumbled.

We survived. As we have worked through turbulent times, much change
has come about: new, clarifying policies; reorganisation toward less hierarchical structures; course offerings on power and control dynamics and
on teaching; explicit focus on a code of conduct; formation of a national

Ombuds-office as a resource for AITs; and encouragement for AITs to belong to and participate in IPSO, including payment of IPSO membership fees by the Institute on behalf of the AITs.

Moving us through this caesura, I feel, was an undercurrent of faith in the psychoanalytic stance. "Investigate the caesura," Bion says, when we are challenged to move from one state of mind to another. "How quickly can we become aware of the changed situation, and how quickly can we see what good use could be made of the changed situation, even though adverse?" (Bion, 1977/2014, p. 44). As turbulent and painful as it was, I felt emboldened to meet the experience, feel it fully, think about it and trust that some use could be made of it. For that, Dear Institute, I thank you.

There has been much to learn, and much to unlearn. Some lessons, Dear Institute, I learned from you. Some I felt I learned despite you. Most lessons I learned with you. One such lesson has been to invite the expression and inclusion of multiple vertices as our Institute continues to evolve and *become*. In fact, our Institute's updated welcome address, developed with the involvement of training analysts, analysts-in-training (AITs) and members of our local psychoanalytic society, now states:

> Our policy will be to re-examine and re-formulate our tenets continually to reflect further creative and imaginative views (aesthetics) arising out of mutual discourse. Each analyst and AIT will influence and determine these aspirations; each analyst and AIT will develop their own personal view and theoretical vertex with the intention of holding a receptive open-door policy to formulate and integrate underlying evolving principles that will inform our Institute.
>
> (WCPSI AIT Orientation Manual Committee, 2023)

With this letter, I would like to join you in this spirit of ongoing examination and reflection. I will begin with some theoretical reflections on play and how it might apply in psychoanalytic education. I will then turn to my personal experience and describe where I felt play worked and where I felt it was hindered during my training. I propose that exploring collapses of play and reorienting toward its creative and prosocial potential could enrich the psychoanalytic learning process.

## Reflections on play in psychoanalytic training

Affective neuroscience research has shown that there are circuits in the brain, common throughout mammalian species, which mediate PLAY (Panksepp, 1998).[2] Beyond its fun and joyful aspects, play offers the opportunity to learn and practice physical as well as social skills. Through play, we experiment and develop ideas. In the psychoanalytic literature, Klein and Winnicott have written extensively about play and its importance for psychic growth and creativity (Klein, 1932/1989; Winnicott, 1971/2017a). It is also through play that we learn our place amongst others in our social structures—where we can win, and where we need to humbly accept losing. Play promotes prosocial thought. Following the 60:40 rule of reciprocity, everyone needs to be given the chance to take the lead some of the time, or they will not want to play anymore (Solms, 2021a).

### Play as an area of learning and practice

Analysts-in-training are, simultaneously, established clinicians yet new learners of psychoanalysis. With regard to the latter, we find ourselves in a *zone of proximal development*, described by psychologist and learning theorist Lev Vygotsky as the distance between the level of what has already been reached and the level of potential development (Vygotsky, 1978). For Vygotsky, play creates a zone of proximal development, in which more advanced functions are tried out, spurring on development. As AITs playing in a zone of proximal development, we need to practice, tumble and fall. We may ask for a hand getting up. At other times, we may want to try it on our own—"Me do it!" We still need your guidance, and the confidence that you will "not fail to be there if suddenly needed" (Winnicott, as cited in Caldwell & Joyce, 2011).

### Play as an area of creativity

The neural PLAY circuits described by Panksepp (1998) include neuroanatomical regions implicated in behavioural switching and set-shifting, leading Kellman and Radwan (2022) to propose that social play may promote the development of flexible, creative adaptations to novelty. Winnicott (1971/2017b) asserts: "It is in playing, and only in playing that the individual child or adult is able to be creative and to use the whole personality, and it is only in being creative that the individual discovers the self" (p. 170).

However, Winnicott alerts us to the impingements from the environment that can inhibit creativity and lead to the development of a false self (Winnicott, 1971/2017a). As an example of such an impingement, he describes: "The patient's creativity can be only too easily stolen by a therapist who knows too much" (Winnicott, 1971/2017b, p. 173). Bion, similarly, cautions against too much knowledge and theory, pointing out in a 1978 seminar at the Tavistock Clinic:

> The noise that those theories make is so great that you can hardly hear yourself think. It is one of these occasions where I think that it is useful to be able to shut off one's awareness of what is going on, so as to get the turmoil cut down enough for some relevant fact to be able to get through.
>
> (Sousa, 2021)

In addition, our play and creativity in psychoanalytic training are shaped by the *hidden curriculum*. Coined by education researcher Philip Jackson (1968), the term hidden curriculum refers to the implicit rules, traditions and expectations that exist along with the 'official' academic curriculum of a learning institution. School success will depend on the mastery of both. Yet Jackson highlights that overly passive conformity to the implicit demands of the institutional setting may be at odds with individual expression and undermine curious probing and exploration (Jackson, 1968).

The need to protect a space for new ideas to emerge amidst the plethora of knowledge and theories we are attempting to take in creates a dilemma. Bion, in his paper *Caesura*, proposes to readers the approach of forgetting the paper, dismissing it from one's mind, unless called into consciousness again by an analysand in the moment of a session (Bion, 1977/2014). Winnicott encourages us to allow for non-purposive, formless states of being, from which creative impulses can arise, which he notes are the "stuff of playing" (Winnicott, 1971/2017b, p. 179). By the same token, we need to remember to play during our studies, to find this unencumbered, creative space. To play Winnicott's squiggle game together, letting go of any preformed pictures and just seeing what might emerge.

### Play as an area of interface with reality

The hallmark of play is laughter. It is associated with joy. It is also socially contagious (Panksepp, 1998). Panksepp puts forth that the positive emotional state generated by play could effectively ease the process of learning. From Winnicott's perspective, the mother's eventual task, after giving sufficient opportunity for illusion, is gradually to disillusion the infant (Winnicott, 1971/2017c). He contends that relief from the strain of reality-acceptance is provided by an intermediate area of experience, which he sees as in direct continuity with the play area of the small child who is 'lost' in play. "If all goes well", he ventures, "the infant can actually come to gain from the experience of frustration" (Winnicott, 1971/2017c, p. 274).

Our psychoanalytic learning includes growing our capacity to receive, hold, contain and co-metabolise painful realities. Bringing in play may help soften the blow. play could easily be romanticised as a fun and joyous way to connect harmoniously with others and put an illusively positive spin on reality. From a neuropsychoanalytic perspective, Solms reminds us that the mammalian PLAY drive is related to establishing hierarchies and testing acceptable limits. Play ceases when these limits are crossed and the 'as if' quality is lost (Solms, 2021b). In puppy play, a playful nip breaks the skin and becomes a serious wound. In larger society, wars break out. And in psychoanalytic institutes?

Imbalances of power and control, ruthless competition for rank and status, unmerciful win-lose dynamics and boundary violations can all signal

PLAY gone terribly wrong. Widening our examination of such phenomena to include considerations of the basic emotion system of PLAY and the needs it is designed to meet may help us—not only by expanding our understanding of these phenomena but also by affording the opportunity to explore how we might reorient toward the prosocial aspects of PLAY. To play successfully, we need to stay within boundaried terrains, take the needs of others into account, balance them with our own and allow space for all players to take the lead at least some of the time.

Getting back to my personal experience, Dear Institute, there were many instances during my training where you kindled play at its best. I entered psychoanalytic training having grown up in a country of conformity. Compliance with convention was explicitly and implicitly valued. Geraniums on the balcony had to be red, not pink. Garbage bags were black, not brown. Any deviations from these implicit rules brought about askew glances. I was once approached by a neighbour, inquiring with concern whether my mother was all right, as she had noticed that the laundry was hung differently on our outdoor hanging rack.[3] On this backdrop, I entered psychoanalytic training with a strong penchant toward following custom. My implicitly held template was a linear process of reading the theory and then dutifully applying it in my clinical practice. When we started reading Freud's texts about the death drive, I was puzzled. I didn't get it. But if Freud said so, it must be true! So, although the concept continued to bewilder me, I bent it and reshaped it in my mind until I found a way to make it somehow fit with what made more inherent sense to me. Only to be flummoxed again when we were assigned readings several months later in which the entire concept of the death drive was toppled. *Now* what was the right answer . . . was there or was there not a death drive?! How freeing it felt when you declared without reserve: "You don't have to agree. Develop your own metapsychology!" I felt encouraged to play and experiment with different ideas and combinations of ideas—and even to imagine and entertain new ones.

At other times, a spirit of play helped round the edges of piercing realities. For example, as I was grappling during a supervision session with a rather stubborn insistence on my part to 'look on the bright side', the following scene from the World War II musical *South Pacific* (Logan, 1958), came to mind:

Navy nurse Nellie, hopelessly optimistic to the point of being called "Knuckle-head Nellie", is looking out over the ocean and gushes:

"Gosh, it's beautiful here! Just look at that yellow sun. And away off in the distance—those lovely little white clouds . . ."

Emile, a hardened-by-life plantation owner who relocated to the South Pacific Island to flee misfortune in his French hometown, replies solemnly:

"Those lovely little white clouds could easily be gunfire."

Nellie's face falls. "Oh, how awful," she sighs.

I described the scene to my supervisor. "That's me and you!" I quipped. We shared a chuckle. The clinical material was still painful, but through this playful interchange in supervision, it stung just a bit less and I felt just a bit more prepared to face the necessary turmoil with my patient.

And yet it is not possible to stay in this bubble. Instances of thwarted play during training could not be avoided. Encounters with the hidden curriculum—with its unspoken but nevertheless subtly transmitted expectations—were inescapable. A raised eyebrow at the choice of a supportive rather than exploratory intervention. Askew glances, reminiscent of those brought about by the pink geraniums long ago, when conference speakers from different schools of thought presented their models. In response, I would find myself prefacing comments with multiple disclaimers. Or feeling tempted to hide any affiliation I felt to certain ideas or approaches entirely.

In the same way that we listen for latent themes underlying the manifest content of a session, or the basic assumptions underlying the activities of a work group, perhaps we can all pay attention to aspects of the hidden curriculum as they inevitably surface, and hold space for creative inquiry. When curricular clashes occur, let's question the status quo, and not get caught up in "this is the way it has always been." As Bion describes when telling the story of a boy who had been referred for difficulty learning mathematics: "You had better listen to this boy doing mathematics, and find out what *his* mathematics are, and what 2 and 2 does add up to" (Sousa, 2021). We need the freedom to play in this regard, to allow for the imaginative discovery of new openings and paths.

The troubled times I mentioned earlier could also be formulated as a collapse of play. Revisiting problematic splits, conflict, power relations, competition and inclusion/exclusion dynamics as reflections of play in disequilibrium may offer additional perspectives to help us expand our exploration, while understanding the emotional needs they are (unsuccessfully) attempting to meet. Our challenge then becomes to reorient toward play's creative and prosocial potential. I say "our" because I believe AITs and training analysts alike have the responsibility to uphold a constructive climate and attend to the well-being of our organisation. We collectively form the Institute.

Naturally, my representation of you, Dear Institute, like any other internal object, will be shaped and coloured by my internal phantasies, although I imagine the collection of letters in this book will reveal a series of common themes. Furthermore, I have focused on ideas around play as I experienced it during my psychoanalytic training, necessarily limiting the scope. The picture remains, therefore, by definition incomplete. Bion (1977/2014) reminds us: "A mountain viewed from different points of the compass *may be* recognisably the same mountain, but it may be such a different view that it appears to be an entirely different mountain" (p. 44).

However, perhaps further thought and conversation may be sparked. Perhaps we can remember that we need to play every once in a while. Not to deny or escape reality, but to dip into realms that will allow us to rehearse new skills. To engage with others and find our place. To access creative thought that may open up new ways of dealing with our realities. To feel joy and excitement at the discovery of new ideas and insights. I hope we can play together and continue this dialogue at conferences and at meetings, through books and within letters.

Amidst the seriousness of our realities, let's keep play alive.

I look forward to seeing you soon!

Sincerely,

— Michelle van den Engh, MD, FRCPC

## Notes

1 Some excerpts from the theoretical reflections and the supervision vignette described in this letter were previously published in a slightly different version in van den Engh, M. (2023). Play in psychoanalytic training: Perks, perils and pivot points. *The Candidate Connection Newsletter of the APSA Candidates' Council*, 25(2), 4–5.

2 In his taxonomy of basic emotion systems, Panksepp (1998) uses uppercase letters to refer to these genetically ingrained operating systems, which include SEEKING, RAGE, FEAR, LUST, PANIC/GRIEF, CARE and PLAY.

3 These are memories of growing up in the German part of Switzerland in the 1980s. Much may have since changed.

# 31 A letter to Société Psychanalytique de Recherche et de Formation, Paris, France (2005)

*Muriel Gayet*

*In France, the psychoanalytic landscape is surprisingly complex. Choosing the institute in which to train as a psychoanalyst leads you to confront a great diversity in training models. And that is not easy to make sense of! The candidate can choose between numerous psychoanalytic societies and schools. Only three of those societies belong to the International Psychoanalytical Association (IPA): the Société Psychanalytique de Paris (SPP, Paris Psychoanalytical Society, 1926), the Association Française de Psychanalyse (APF, French Psychoanalytical Association, 1964) and the Société Psychanalytique de Recherche et de Formation (SPRF, Psychoanalytical Society for Research and Training, 2005). In a historically centralized country, most of these Institutes are located in Paris and offer their own variation of the IPA French model.*

*There are many other psychoanalytic societies. Most of them claim to be descending from the teachings of Lacan, to a greater or a lesser extent. They train a large number of psychoanalysts according to varied training paths, throughout the country.*

*Within the SPRF, training is following the IPA French model. It is structured around two consecutive individual supervisions, two clinical seminars lasting for two years each, and a range of courses and seminars that you can freely choose from, whereas the Eitingon model offers a scheduled series of seminars over a period of four or five years. It isn't an entirely individual process either, unlike with the Quatrième groupe (Fourth Group), which the SPRF split from. The SPRF is a rather young psychoanalytic Society and we don't have an Institute as such. However, for the sake of standardization, I have used the phrase "Dear Institute" throughout this letter.*

*The training process relies on a dual process of inputs by the society, and the necessary appropriation brought by the candidate in their individual approach. Two consecutive supervised cases must be approved by an evaluating group composed of teaching analysts selected at random. They focus on the way the presenting candidate appropriated the process of supervision. The supervisor also reports on that on their own. Once the two supervisions are approved, candidates have to write a theoretical and clinical text that will then be presented and discussed with an ad-hoc training committee in order to complete the training and qualify as a member.*

DOI: 10.4324/9781003465409-31

*I would like to thank warmly the editor who dared to imagine such a book, echoing* Dear Candidate, *which I had a fantastic time reading. This initiative demonstrates the ability to gather multiple candidates of various backgrounds for a brave and innovative project. It gives us the opportunity to present our thoughts on this topic, and deepen our gaze into our training in progress. Writing this contribution has been inspiring. I thought about the dozens of colleagues working on the same topic all around the globe, and I am eager to read what they came up with and to discover the diversity of our paths.*

—

So, why did I choose you, dear Institute, to train me?

When I decided to become an analyst, which was driven by my personal experience as an analysand, I knew very little about the psychoanalytic societies in France. At that time, in 2008, I came from a very different world, since I was working in the corporate sector, after a scientific postgraduate degree. I knew that I wanted to work in private practice as well as within a mental health institution, to carry on the kind of multidisciplinary teamwork that I had greatly appreciated in my professional life so far.

During my years studying psychology in college, I wandered around the open activities of various psychoanalytic societies that I was hearing about, without finding the right place. Choosing an institute is a process in itself as well as a long-term decision, since you will stay with the same people long after the training is finished.

When I started practicing psychology, in the psychiatric department of a public hospital, I asked a colleague whose clinical skills I admired to refer me to a supervisor, in order to be supported for the first steps of my career. She directed me towards a teaching analyst at the SPRF, where she herself was in training.

During my encounters with that analyst, who then became the supervisor of my first case, the aim was to improve how I was analytically listening to the psychotic patients of the outpatient center, but also to reflect on *becoming an analyst*. Our initial exchange led to long and fruitful work regarding listening, setting, ethics, as well as the stakes of the various training models and psychoanalytic branches, all within the context of the history of psychoanalysis in France and other countries . . . This axis of research greatly enriched my training, which officially began two years later, when I applied to be a candidate at the SPRF.

My first steps with you, dear Institute, were somewhat intimidating, especially during seminars, which gathered members and candidates for theoretical and clinical presentations related to a yearly theme. Back then, the SPRF was a Study Group that later became a Component Society in 2015. The process of being recognized by the IPA was applying pressure on you as a young society that had to prove itself. Belonging to the IPA was an important issue for the founding members, who left the *Quatrième Groupe* following disagreements on the training process, which they believed to be too vague. Instead, they wanted to get closer to the international dynamic of the IPA. Obtaining the status of Component Society was an important institutional step, as well as a source of pride and relief.

I quickly got involved in theoretical seminars and a clinical seminar, while progressing into the first supervision. I had so much to learn with so many questions arising in me. Would I be able to go through this long training? How to prioritize my readings? Sometimes, in order to help me understand specific points, my supervisor drew parallels with his own patients. I remember that when I was leaving his practice, I sometimes still did not clearly see what he wanted me to understand even though I was feeling an unconscious resonance. It often made sense afterwards and sometimes following a significant delay. Dear Institute, I am so grateful for this thought-provoking experience that continues to help me in my daily practice. When my first supervised case was approved after five years, I remember realizing how much I had grown. This step was an encouragement and gave me the impulse to take a role of IPSO. I also became more active in my training. For example, I was struggling to find group supervision regarding my practice involving psychotic patients, which was also the case for a colleague of mine. We ended up running a study group on psychosis together.

When the Covid-19 pandemic started in March 2020, training moved online. In-person encounters were suddenly impossible due to the lockdown put in place by the French government, like in many other countries. Relationships within the SPRF analytic community were strained by not being together before, after, and during seminars. We didn't have those informal moments during which we could talk among ourselves, even though we needed it even more than usual. Luckily, dear Institute, you created support groups to give us some space to share feelings and try to figure out what was happening in the world and in our own lives. Each group set its online meeting frequency and the way it was run. This was very helpful during those first few months. At the same time, new opportunities were created to attend online seminars and conferences across continents, making me feel as if unexpected doors were opening. Some candidates from our Institute also decided to gather in the same place to watch the 2021 European Psychoanalytical Federation (EPF) conference together. I remember this moment as a unique opportunity to spend some good time together. It helped us to wait for the next in-person conference in Vienna.

Video conferences and phone sessions took a major place in my analytic life at that time. I switched to sessions over the phone as an analysand, a supervisee, and both in clinic and private practice. I think that it was of great interest to experience phone sessions as an analysand. It helped me figure out what this unusual setting was inducing on both sides, whereas remote analysis was until then a big taboo for French psychoanalysts. In supervision, I sometimes felt lonely being far from my supervisor's place, but there were also surprising moments of increased intimacy, despite the distance. I was relieved when supervision could finally take place in-person again.

Since my second supervision is now finished, dear Institute, it seems to me that supervisions are at the heart of my training process. In addition to a focus on transference and countertransference, maintaining the frame and formulating interpretations, there is also a focus on my own transfer on the supervision and the institution. This makes supervision a rich thinking space. I also find it fruitful that both candidate and supervisor can share their own thoughts with the evaluating group. This process has been established as an attempt to limit the effects of alienation during supervision, even if it cannot accomplish that goal on its own. Candidates can also meet two teaching analysts dedicated to help one get out of a dead end during the training process. We can encounter them during group meetings and individual appointments, an initiative that is often taken by candidates approaching an important or challenging step during training. This opportunity is used by some of us, while others do not think to or dare to do it.

Any psychoanalytic society faces institutional issues and may be threatened by the insidious risks of subjection and alienation throughout the training process. The study of this concern was pioneered by the *Quatrième Groupe*. Our society has tried to pay attention to that concern in order to avoid falling back into a pattern of violence flowing from the previous generations of analysts to the next. Nevertheless, dear Institute, there is no perfect solution to avoid these underlying risks. Our numbers are still small enough to enable us to gather members and candidates in one room for group discussion. Those meetings, held once or twice a year, can be tense and frustrating, but allow for valuable group work by both candidates and members, similar to an institutional meeting. This task will always remain incomplete, but it is deeply useful, and I believe it to be a real strength of our institution.

Throughout my training, I have had mixed feelings regarding your size, dear Institute. With a current average of 20 members and 30 candidates, training takes place in an atmosphere of collegiality which means a lot to us. It offers individual space for everyone and a valuable diversity of theoretical and clinical orientations, despite a limited number of teaching analysts and seminars. We are supposed to complete our training by exploring outside of its bounds. I gradually understood that I shouldn't only rely on the SPRF. Instead, it functions as a set of foundations, aiming at being a *good enough* institution.

I still think that a psychoanalytic approach to groups and institutions would be useful for all of us, especially those working within teams. A familiarity with these concepts would also enable us to understand more precisely group dynamics in the Institute. During EPF conferences, I am therefore particularly interested in presentations on institutions, as well as in some exciting workshops, among which "Workshop on the Specificity of Psychoanalytical Treatment Today" and the "Large Group", the latter capturing the broader scope of societal history and dynamics.

Due to our size, dear Institute, we also share an underlying concern about our long-term development. Despite the huge work done since 2005 to give shape to our society, the SPRF still has little visibility and is barely represented in universities and conferences. This makes it sometimes difficult to attract new candidates for training. The generation of founding members, who were all experienced analysts in 2005, are gradually passing the baton. Some growth would better distribute the institutional work and the investment in the local and international scientific community.

Our society is however attracting candidates who are interested in its multicultural and international aspects, and in a shared responsibility regarding a rigorous and flexible training, without the need to belong to a long-established society. Some of us speak multiple languages, some have multicultural backgrounds, and some have even lived abroad. Unlike most candidates in other French societies, we are significantly involved in international events organized by IPSO.

IPSO is adding so much to my training journey! This is why I decided to take part in this book, so I could share my experiences.

We aim to introduce IPSO to new candidates as soon as they join us, dear Institute, so that they benefit from this dynamic from the start of their training. Members also warmly encourage candidates to get involved with IPSO, despite the fact that most of them, who trained outside the IPA, did not have this opportunity during their own training.

IPSO brings people together in many ways. The clinical study group I have been a part of for three years is one of my best psychoanalytical experiences! This unique space allows close friendships to grow between people living all over the globe. Those friendships provide invaluable support, especially regarding doubts and inhibitions about our supervised cases, questions and excitement about writing and presenting at conferences, as well as new perspectives and new goals once we become members. We also discuss how societal and political events occurring in our respective countries and around the world affect us, as analysts and citizens.

In addition to international connections, IPSO facilitates relationships and initiatives between candidates belonging to the three French societies, such as working together to organize international scientific IPSO events in Paris.

IPSO also strengthens the bonds between candidates from our own Institute by giving us the opportunity to live exciting moments abroad that create lasting memories throughout a training period that can last for a long time within the French model.

In the French model, training takes place at a less intensive pace than in the Eitingon model, as well as in a more individualized way. Our fellow candidates following the Eitingon model start out younger, they have not been in analysis for as long, and they become members more quickly than us. That latter point can sometimes awaken envy within us, with similar feelings towards the college student atmosphere of the cohort. However, we do appreciate the separation between our personal analysis and our training, as well as the freedom we are granted when it comes to picking our lectures and seminars.

In our training process, the five to eight years usually needed for the two supervisions to be approved are followed by the highly transformative last part of the training: writing and presenting a theoretical and clinical paper. This phase which I have just entered, dear Institute, is often experienced as a solitary and initiatory in-between. The process of writing is arduous for some of us: pleasure, pain, even torture . . . All kinds of fantasies surround writing and presenting. At that stage, some candidates find it useful to share their struggles and help each other within an informal group of peers.

Becoming a member is at stake, which induces an identity adjustment that spares no one. It can take years for some people to get beyond that point, and some never even succeed. Their two supervised cases are approved, but they do not become members, when candidates from some other IPA societies qualify as associate members as soon as their second supervised case is approved. The risk inherent in this system, underlined in our lively discussions on this subject, would be to remain an associate member, which would prevent one from taking a mutative step in being an analyst and becoming more involved in their respective society.

So, dear Institute, what is gained and what is lost by becoming a member? Beyond personal stakes, the institutional stakes vary from one society to the next. In some of the older societies, recent members are not engaged much, or they struggle to find ways to get involved, since the older, established generations seem to leave no empty spots. In our case, becoming a member means getting your voice heard and quickly being expected to contribute. This perspective might add more mixed feelings. Will I be able to say goodbye to my candidate status, to IPSO, and find how to take part in my own way as a member in the institutional life and in the psychoanalytic community?

Thank you, my dear Institute, and thank you also to the previous generations who, one after another, contributed to the transmission of psychoanalysis. Let's hope that we will be able, in our turn, to train the next generations, taking into account the unprecedented challenges of our time.

— Muriel Gayet

# 32 A letter to Instituto Latinoamericano de Psychoanalysis, Guatemala City, Guatemala (2006)

*Liza M. Zachrisson*

*ILAP (The Latin American Institute of Psychoanalysis) is a relatively recent project of the IPA and FEPAL. Its formal origin, marked by the signature of a memorandum recording an agreement between the presidents of both institutions, Claudio Eizirik and Alvaro Rey de Castro respectively, dates from January 2006, but the governing body of ILAP was formed in December of the same year (García, 2011).*

*Guatemala is a country with no Psychoanalytic association nor trained analysts, so in 2015 a group of psychologists from Guatemala, myself included, attended the IPA Boston congress, where we were introduced to ILAP, an institute created by FEPAL and IPA, that enables people who live in Latin-American countries with no training institutes nor IPA associations to train as psychoanalysts. Before the pandemic, the training in ILAP was through condensed analysis where one week a month, to meet the 100-hour required per year, the analyst-in-training would travel to the training analyst's country and would have two daily sessions to complete approximately ten sessions each visit. Supervisions required two high frequency analysis to be supervised by two different analysts, completing 80 hours of supervisions, with 30% of them being in person. Seminars were also condensed; each seminar was given over two to three continuous days. Since the pandemic started, seminars, supervisions, and training analysis were allowed virtually, which permitted the condensed part to be taken out, and seminars became weekly classes given throughout a semester with all ILAP candidates from different countries in Central America (Guatemala, Honduras, Nicaragua, El Salvador), and some countries in South America (Ecuador, Bolivia). In addition to this, training analysis became three or more sessions a week every week. All seminars, supervisions, and training analyses were given by training analysts who were members of other IPA associations from different countries in Latin America.*

*After meeting ILAP in Boston, we organized three different academic activities throughout a five-year period, where we did two-to-three-day conferences. ILAP directives would come to Guatemala, and we got to know each other. This relationship lasted about five years. A year after joining the training, ILAP's directives changed abruptly. An email was sent that the entire directive would change, and a meeting was called with all training analysts to be*

DOI: 10.4324/9781003465409-32

*introduced to the new directive. Shortly after, they announced changes being made to the curriculum, duration and evaluation process of the seminars.*

—

Dear ILAP:

Living in a country where psychoanalysis is something you read about in books and talk about but don't have a place, a group, an institution that enables you to train as a psychoanalyst, is a complex experience that feels like there are many obstacles and challenges along the path. Living in Guatemala and having the desire to become a psychoanalyst has felt that way. Since my first years studying psychology in university, the desire to know and understand more about psychoanalysis awoke, and with that, the frustration of not having a place to learn and understand such a complex theory and way of working with patients. For many years it felt like a wish that would not be fulfilled because moving or traveling to another country to train as a psychoanalyst meant leaving behind my clinical practice that had taken so much time to build. The more time passed, the harder it felt to move away from my practice. So, I decided to participate in what was possible and at reach. I enrolled in online seminars given by analysts in other associations, organized virtual academic activities, and created with a couple of colleagues a space to think and write about psychoanalysis. In 2015, when I was introduced to you during the Boston IPA congress, at first it felt like a surreal opportunity – to finally have a possibility to train to become a psychoanalyst. It also felt very challenging because although training finally became an option, it was a complicated one. I felt the frequency of the condensed analysis wasn't thinking so much about the candidates process in analysis and the consistency one needs from an analyst's presence as a patient, rather it felt like it was more about fulfilling your desires and requirements than my needs as a patient. When this option was first presented to me I was starting my first pregnancy and having condensed periods of time to be so absent from my baby felt conflicting, even contradictory to what psychoanalysis proposes for a mothers presence. So although the opportunity you presented was there, the timing for me wasn't. When the pandemic came, and your conditions changed, I felt like an opportunity was raised: a sustainable way to start the training where I could have a high frequency analysis in a consistent format that was more like the "real" traditional format that other candidates have with multiple weekly sessions and, weekly seminars that would enabled me to digest the content for the seminars week by week, as well as the material in my own analysis. To have my training analysis in a much similar way to what was intended felt opportune, not to fulfill your requisite, but to feel contained and held by an institution and an analyst in the way it should be. Fortunately, you, the timing, my desire, and technology all came together for the opportunity to begin a virtual and more consistent training for an uncertain period of time. And so, my so longed desire of becoming a psychoanalyst finally started coming true.

Because you give this training opportunity to candidates from different countries of Latin America, we are all united by the same language but with its particularities of how we each use this language. With a common Latin culture, that has similar political and social dynamics, and different contexts. We are all united in a virtual meeting room ("many floating heads" as an analyst one said during a seminar), it feels comforting to be united with colleagues that share our passion and desire to become a psychoanalyst in a country where training feels lonely at times. I also feel understood by my fellow candidates that also have faced similar obstacles to begin the training. It's not the same when we talk with candidates from an institute that already exists in their country, because all though similarities exist, the differences can't be denied. But in this meeting room we are all together, in different countries with similar obstacles, poor third world countries were social and economical and political conflicts constantly shake our societies, but because we don't live in the same one, they don't happen at the same time or in the same way, so there is a sense of holding and containment that we give each other when corruption scandals brake and environmental disasters hit. This gives a sense of community that feels comforting and close. Our timings are different, but our struggles are similar, with much more similarity than from other countries of South America, North America, or Europe. All though we have not yet met in person, the representation of a group of colleagues that train together and hold each other exists.

In the same way that having a diverse group of candidates has been such an enriching experience, having a diverse group of analysts dictating seminars, as well as supervisors and analysts also feels enriching, giving us the exposure to how different parts of Latin America think, talk and are traversed by psychoanalysis. It gives us a wonderful tasting of how psychoanalytic associations work and how that exposure impacts us when we are the ones who build our countries association from the ground up after we become IPA psychoanalysts. It feels similar to a kid looking at parents and fantasying on how it will be when you're the adult, to learn a part of what has already been built in other places and in different places.

Because you are not a place, but an institute without walls and rooms, you are the most abstract representation of an institution. You exist in word, in presence, but not in a place so the transference is to the directors, because you are only conformed by directors and training analysts. When we began our relationship with you and your directives, before starting the training, the change from one directive to the other felt like there was a continuing, a legacy that was passed on from one to the other and that helped me decide to join an institute without walls, because I had met it's representatives through the years and through that we had built a relationship with you. However, a couple of months after joining the training there was an abrupt (and what felt like a) violent change when all your directives had to leave without notice or any information for us to process this change. A whole new directive came, along with many changes to the training, and although many of those changes now feel like positive ones, the abruptness of this felt like an earthquake that shakes the ground of a building that isn't even built yet. I imagine there was a big conflict within you and your superiors when that change happened, I fantasize that because of that conflict your change was never properly addressed or explained, and that felt very difficult, especially because there was no one and nowhere to come to. IPA, FEPAL, and Organización de Candidatos de América Latina (OCAL) felt so far away. This shake brought positive changes to the training, but it definitely felt it was done in a sudden, unexplained, dramatic move. I remember a fellow candidate describing it so well: "it feels like being caught in the middle of a shooting" (unfortunately a common situation in our countries), but a silent one. Fortunately, we had our analysts outside of ILAP, and each other to process these changes. Although that moment felt difficult, and even unnamable with you, good changes came with it, but it took time and sessions to process and elaborate.

Since the pandemic, before and after I joined the training, I've heard in so many webinars and discussion panels, analysts talk and question the virtual psychoanalysis of training analysts. When training analysts from other institutes ask me how it feels to analyze only virtually, I don't have a point of comparison because I started the training this way. But, having this be the only experience I've had, I can honestly say the psychoanalytic function transcends a screen, the talking cure is abstract, if flows through words, and a presence that exists beyond a body's presence. When I hear discussions about leaving this option closed and returning to only in person sessions for the training, I feel that for your candidates it will be a step back. I can imagine there certainly must be many differences from walking in an analyst's office, laying in their divan, and knowing they are physically there; an experience I very much look forward to living, however, in your situation, I strongly believe this option of having three or more virtual sessions weekly feels a lot closer to a psychoanalytic process, than going back to condensed analysis and condensed seminars. Virtuality is a tool and an obstacle, but for us it became an opportunity. One that has led to you gaining many new candidates in such a short time. Knowing this debate is still up for discussion among IPA directives, some who perhaps haven't had to train under your pre-pandemic requirements is difficult, it continues to feel like a constant shake. I guess being a part of you means having constant shakes. And within those shakes, it feels comforting to be able to identify with an analyst, a teacher, a supervisor that has had a similar experience of training without an institute in their hometown or country. Having that in my own analysis definitely felt important for my process, and it was necessary when I joined you to have someone with a similar training experience and a similar culture to feel understood in its complexities. Part of the training experience and process is identification, I think that is something that takes place in the transference with the analyst, with the supervisor, with fellow candidates, and it should also take place with you.

Psychoanalytic training definitely requires a lot of time and energy but most of all an intense desire to form, emotionally and academically, to question yourself, your theories, your experiences, your background. It is a full-on process that does transform you in amazing ways, with incredible obstacles, challenges, and opportunities. So much that I would have probably missed if you didn't exist. So, dear institute – thank you, you have given me an opportunity to train in something I'm passionate about, learn, evolve, through the seminars, my own analysis, and supervisions; you have exposed me to such a diverse world that exists within IPA that I only imagined, and that being a part of it is much more complex, demanding and exciting than what I imagined it to be. And although it sometimes feels like building a city where there is nothing around, you have given me a community abroad, tools, and so much more to do so. I look forward to continue training with you and one day be part of the group of founders that builds the first IPA association and training institute in Guatemala.

With warm regards,

— Liza M. Zachrisson

# 33 A letter to the Istanbul Psychoanalytical Association, Turkey (2007)

*Huner Aydin*

*As a relatively young association, Istanbul Psychoanalytical Association was founded in 2001. In January 2007 four founder members of this association constituted the 'Turkish Psychoanalytical Study Group' recognized by the board of the IPA. Then it was promoted to Provisional Study status in 2013 and became a 'Component Society' in 2017. Currently there are 50 psychoanalysts, and 110 candidates having training.*

*In order to be qualified as a psychoanalyst in our institution, two supervision cases must continue for at least two years. One of these supervisions can be done outside the institution, with an IPA member Training Analyst. Many candidates receive supervision from Training Analysts from different countries. This gives the opportunity to get acquainted with different psychoanalytic schools and tendencies. To become a psychoanalyst, it is also necessary to attend at least three theoretical seminars and at least one clinical seminar for two years. For the formation completion interview, one of these two supervision cases must be presented.*

—

Dear Institute,

'I have never thought that psychoanalysis is such an impossible work', I guess that would be the phrase that best describes my current emotions. I had always found theories of various psychotherapy training I had taken throughout years of my psychiatry practice on the human mind superficial. That had always led me to research on deeper and hidden aspects of the human mind. I thought that psychoanalysis was the right address to do so, but it seemed that it wasn't accessible for me, both physically and emotionally. When I started my own analysis, I had no thoughts about being a psychoanalyst, it was still somewhere far away. After some months I decided to become an analyst, probably my identification with my analyst made it possible for me. That's how I started having a training in psychoanalysis after a tedious application process.

Psychoanalysis training is very valuable and special, but it is a process that also entails lots of frustration. A hovering 'grief' accompanies you in the next

DOI: 10.4324/9781003465409-33

step, or the frustration of not being able to take the next step. Over the years, the lost 'innocence' accompanied by vanishing idealizations gives way to a confusion called 'growth', which brings emotional maturation and transformation as much as unmet expectations leading you to opposite directions. Those unmet expectations are always accompanied with various reveries. Such thoughts as 'that training analyst seems to be closer to that candidate', 'they don't think I am bright enough' linger in the mind. Having or not having the consent to accept the first patient on the couch or not being able to find a suitable patient while enthusiastically anticipating your first patient might bring about frustration and hard feelings. It gets more and more difficult to cope with the frustration of your empty couch when candidates in your group one by one start to talk about their analysands. After passing this step then you need to cope with the anxiety at the back of your mind about the prospects of your patient giving up the analysis, while curiously receiving all that is about your first case with great interest. My impression from other candidates is that it can be a really traumatic experience to have your first patient quitting the analysis at some point. A hidden anger against the patient or the supervisor is the accompanying feeling when the process doesn't work out. The feeling that you cannot 'progress', stagnancy and lack of motivation accompanying this anger.

The confusion that comes along with new concepts successively rushing in our minds during intense seminar programs leads to the expectation that a good training analyst with a more satisfying knowledge could explicate things better, but that analyst is nowhere to be found. You frequently feel like it is 'impossible' for all those concepts to become integrated. The fact that these trainers interpret these concepts differently along with different discourses regarding the institutional structure and organization sometimes create more confusion. Not knowing which one to trust and follow somehow leads you to accept that psychoanalysis is part of the human condition and it lacks certainty. Of course this acceptance comes 'years later'.

Over the years, a feeling of inadequacy appeared in me as to why I hadn't yet developed my own ideas. Needless to say, I had been to various seminars, I had read and discussed a lot, then why couldn't I feel myself more authentic and productive! Only years later could I finally tolerate the feeling of inadequacy and inefficacy accompanied by the feeling of not having enough experience or knowledge and accept that it took a lot of time to develop one's own theory. Although it is part of the training to learn how to trust in one's own intuition and the work of her own unconscious; not to know where to go in between tons of concepts, theories, supervisor attitudes; feeling perturbed in all the steps, in fact, my own unconscious has indeed told me what to do from the beginning. In the end, analysis is also an art and the artist relies on her unconscious to nurture her creativity.

Another thing which emerges during the period of candidacy, which goes hand in hand with the feeling of inadequacy, is the desire that you will be better than your analyst, supervisor and many others in the future. The phantasy is 'some analysts and training analysts have not managed to be good enough, but we will not be like them in the future!' The institution is separated into good analysts and trainers and bad analysts and trainers and you desire to meet and work with the 'good' ones during your candidacy. When one gets disappointed also by the 'good' ones, then you start to question the value of psychoanalysis. An intense candidacy period accompanied by all those splitting, idealization and identification constitutes the building block of your emotional growth. It is not always easy to tolerate 'a constant state of uncertainty', and peer support might then be the most urgent intervention. On the other hand, although we are surrounded with individual analysis, peer groups and supervision, there is the lingering feeling of how lonely we are in reality.

My analysis was hard from time to time. I could barely speak on the couch for the first two months, I felt like my analyst vanished into thin air. I remembered the challenges in my own analysis when I started to receive analysands on the couch. I was surprised to see how comfortably my analysands were talking. The patience of my analyst was also surprising. Now I realize that I internalized my analyst's patience. It is interesting to see that my analysands are very talkative! My first two analysands talked about their dreams in almost all sessions. I had the same expectation from my third analysand, but things were different this time. I realized that I had to learn being an analyst anew with each analysand.

My training coincided with a time in which psychoanalysis practice in the world was going through rapid transformations. The emergence of online work with the pandemic will undoubtedly substantially affect our practice in the upcoming years. This led to a radical change in our perception of the relationship between time and space which are the essentials of psychoanalysis. In a time when we were in the process of learning which theories and concepts to lean on, concepts regarding the foundations of psychoanalytical relationship became controversial, which made the ground of our practice more slippery.

Although the seminars sparked enthusiasm at the beginning, I sometimes lost this excitement and interest in a short span of time. I think I was expecting the conditions to be more active and livelier. In time, I realized that this also had a transferential aspect. This is the frustration created by parents who do not respond to their kid's excitement with a similar enthusiasm. Each seminar has a unique character. In some of them, it is mostly the moderator who talks, some others are more interactive and we make close reading of articles in others. The fact that these seminars are not standardized makes us exposed to different experiences and it matches well with the individualizing spirit of psychoanalysis. The moderator chooses the reading materials in the seminars, and it is for sure important to not restrict oneself to the reading material. There is a huge literature and amazing authors out there. I was at a loss as to the scope of this literature, but it helped me keep my courage to start with the more accessible and easy-to-read ones. We were lucky that our institution had a flexible attitude towards teaching different approaches and theories.

Not feeling obliged to adopt a single approach makes room for freedom and creativity.

Dear institute – I would like to request that you keep this approach alive, even if this flexibility creates various tensions in the psychoanalytical institution.

The presence of supervisors, a significant leg of the training, also created some challenges. Above all, do we listen to the patient to understand him/her or to show the supervisor how accurate our remarks are? Or do we listen to them to credit or discredit certain psychoanalytical concepts? We listen to them sometimes for one or all of the above reasons. When I am working with control cases, I both deeply need the presence of a third party, the supervisor, but at the same time I want to get him/her out of the room immediately. The relationship with the supervisor can thus be complicated. Being able to manage this relationship was for sure part of our growth. What to do when we disagree with him/her? Will we express it openly or complete the process without getting into a conflict with him/her?! Knowing that the supervisor, as a parent and authority figure, has the potential to reveal the complex feelings our need for him/her creates, how to continue this relationship?! For that very reason, many candidates tend to choose supervisors they get along with or deem 'good-tempered'.

Dear institute, although I am so grateful to you for so much, I wish there was a bit more guidance from you on how to navigate the complexities of the supervisory relationship.

We attend seminars in different groups in the unique education model of our institution so we could attend the same seminars with candidates from lower or higher groups. It gave us the opportunity to meet with other candidates and discuss with candidates having different levels of experience. All candidate groups also conducted a number of meetings and corporate and clinical studies with two analysts, supervisors outside the institution once a year. The chance to work with trainers from different countries with various institutional backgrounds was also a very enriching experience. The group got very excited each time when we started the effort to make research on who to work with and contact them. Supervisors from various countries such as France, Greece, Israel, Germany sparked curiosity. It created both tension and excitement to make psychoanalytical work with a supervisor I had never seen before in a foreign language. This 'foreign' supervisor also didn't know what to expect; similarly, s/he was also about to work with candidates from a different culture who s/he never met before. Perhaps, s/he was going to be somehow tested by us. Idealizing these foreign supervisors is a dominant feeling in the group, as they come from a century-old psychoanalysis practice and know-how, while we are in the process of institutionalizing psychoanalysis in a young institution. These 'foreign' supervisors were curiously awaited each time with great interest, while the 'insiders' had already become familiar and lost their charm.

'Experiential Reflective Group' work with Yossi Triest, an Israeli training analyst, which lasted for five years and in which I had the chance to work on group unconscious, was among the trainings which contributed to the development of my own psychoanalytical notion during the training process. Yossi Triest was also a supervisor who visited our association to give training. Upon his suggestion to conduct an experiential group work in a time when he was with us for a training, I had excitedly made my application. We were 12 candidates to meet three times a year. I had wondered how I could open myself up in front of other candidates in this group work which I attended with great anxiety, not knowing what to expect! Yossi had a theme called 'being an analyst in difficult times'. Our country was politically going through turbulent times at that period and ISIS used to conduct bomb attacks frequently. Yossi's theme was really what we needed. In the first meetings, we tried somehow not to reveal our unconscious material, as if this can be possible. Some left the group a year later and we continued to work with the remaining seven people for four years.

In this group study, we used Bion's concepts on group psychodynamics. There were seven female participants and a male group leader. This led to the emergence of intense transferential feelings. Who would be chosen amongst us by this father, lover, mother figure to be his favorite! Who would be the most brilliant one! Anxiety and conflicting emotions appeared at the background of this theme about being a psychoanalyst in difficult times. As seven women, how close or distant we were to be with the male leader and among each other! How far would we go to compete! We were to continue with those female candidates in the same seminars, supervisors or maybe on the couch with same analyst after experiencing conflictual emotions in this group. Therefore, how would we allow ourselves to meet with our truth in this group work! We were lucky to have an experienced container. Thanks to him, we could proceed to become a 'work group' in years.

I went through a meaningful experience which would enlighten me about group interactions as a member of a psychoanalytical association in the largest sense of the word within different groups, peer supervision, seminar groups. Whenever I am in a group, I go out of the situation in my mind and zoom in Yossi's remarks. The unanswered questions I have about not having or even avoiding group work in psychoanalytical institutions come to my mind.

In recent years, many colleagues have been applying to our organization to start the formation process. However, the relatively small number of education analysts may cause the duration of supervision to be limited to the formal duration of two years. In reality, this is not enough time for a supervision work to be sufficiently internalized. Here the pressure from external reality tries to accelerate the 'sufficient time' required for an analytical work. Again, many congresses, symposiums and conferences are organized in our institution every year. The contribution of this to education and institutional life is of course undeniable, but this situation also brings along a situation of being too busy with external reality.

And then there is IPSO, of course! It was such an exciting experience. It was such a chance to have the opportunity to meet with candidates from around the world and share experiences. It was as if the world got smaller and there was psychoanalysis everywhere. Talking with candidates from other countries, it was both surprising and curious to see how each psychoanalytical institution was both similar and different. On the other hand, it was also comforting to see that many candidates dealt with similar problems. That feeling went hand in hand with a sense of confrontation and questioning your own institution.

In writing this letter, I was getting prepared to complete my training, which brings about other intense feelings. Getting ready to say farewell to being a candidate, I wonder whether I have enough qualifications to become an analyst. Have I managed to develop my own concepts to serve me as the foundation of my own practice while I was getting through the intense knowledge I was exposed to about psychoanalytical theories and concepts! The freedom of listening to the analyst without the presence of a supervisor in the meeting room goes hand in hand with doubts about whether I make the correct remarks or not. I have finally become an analyst after months of report-writing. I wonder whether 'is everything starting now!'

— Huner Aydin

# 34 A letter to the Korean Institute for Psychoanalysis, Seoul (2007)

*Chang Jeung Park*

*History of Psychoanalysis in Korea and KIPSA (Korean Institute for Psychoanalysis).*

    *The history of psychoanalysis in Korea began in 1980 and was headed by Dr. Doo Young Cho. As the Sigourney Award winner in 2003, he has made a tremendous contribution to the advancement of psychoanalysis in Korea. Serving then as a professor at the Department of Neuropsychiatry, Seoul National University Hospital, Dr. Cho organized the Seoul Psychoanalysis Research Group, consisting of five psychiatrists who started having a regular psychoanalysis meeting every Wednesday. Instead of conducting psychoanalysis, they performed psychoanalytic psychotherapy and studied psychoanalysis one or two times a week. With their passion and interest in psychoanalysis, this gathering grew rapidly. In 1990, this group changed its name to the Korean Association of Psychoanalysis (KAPA). KAPA was an organization made up of psychiatrists only and was not an institute that could train psychoanalysts. Eventually, KAPA launched the Korean Psychoanalysis Study Group (KPSG) in 2007, which provided psychoanalysis education and initiated a psychoanalyst training program under certification of the IPA, until around 2017, when KPSG ran into conflict with the IPA concerning its policies, specifically, the "non-discrimination policy"—meaning that a psychoanalyst training institute must be an organization where not only psychiatrists but also all mental health professionals can join. The IPA had adhered to this policy, which meant any organization not following such guide would have hard time providing psychoanalyst training programs in Korea. Consequently, launch of new psychoanalyst training programs in Korea came to a halt and there had been disagreements and conflicts among members during the process of accepting this policy as suited to the Korean culture. After going through a series of democratic procedures, the KPSG acceded to the IPA policy, though with some analysts leaving the group. KPSG resumed its analyst training program in 2020 after changing its official name to KIPSA. Since KIPSA and KAPA had different objectives, KIPSA broke away from KAPA as an independent organization. The KIPSA then acquired a provisional society status, becoming an institute that freely performs all functions and provides education independently. It*

DOI: 10.4324/9781003465409-34

*was during this time of change that I joined the journey of my psychoanalyst training in Korea.*

—

Dear Institute,

When I was asked to write this letter, I had a vague fear. Even though it was a welcome suggestion, revealing my story was something difficult for me personally, as an individual who may be under the influence of both the oedipal issue and the Eastern culture. I unconsciously wanted to avoid it but finally made it after going through many revisions. I decided to write this letter to tell you how psychoanalysis in Korea is dynamically changing nowadays. At this point, I was convinced that sharing my thoughts as a candidate with the KIPSA as well as other cultural institutes would be helpful to both KIPSA and myself.

I would like to begin by telling you what I experienced at the beginning of my psychoanalyst candidate training. When I decided to join the training course (2019–2020) at then KPSG, there were still conflicts over the issue of accepting the IPA's non-discrimination policy, which had been around since 2017. In KPSG, there was no psychoanalyst or candidate with a professional mental health background, other than psychiatrists, which led to a delayed start of my training even after my admission until another mental health professional was admitted. My training was suspended for more than a year. Meanwhile, there were emerging political conflicts between two groups within the KPSG—one group trying to accept the IPA's non-discrimination policy and the other group thinking the concept did not fit in the Korean culture. Since our training had not even started, we could not help but just watch the process with bated breath, having no chance to speak. As candidates, we were left feeling helpless and anxious. Being a member of KAPA at the time, I was used to working with psychiatrists only so the whole situation made me confused and conflicted. While I was struggling with the issue, I realized that this has already happened in the history of psychoanalysis in the United States, Europe and other countries. Through case studies of other countries, I found out that non-discrimination policies are linked to the basic principles of psychoanalysis and despite the concerns, they bring quite a lot of benefits. At the end, I came to agree with the non-discrimination policy, and became positive about accepting not only psychiatrists but also other mental health professionals as psychoanalytic trainees. My confusion was gradually resolved; however, the conflict exploded within the KPSG. The group opposing the policy superficially claimed that it was difficult to accommodate the concept due to the specificity of the Korean culture. I thought this claim was rather political than following the basic principle of psychoanalysis. Of course, everyone has their own opinion and I respect it. I also understood that KPSG and KAPA could not go together when they had different goals.

After all the struggles and conflict-settling efforts, KPSG finally decided to accept the IPA's non-discrimination policy and our training could begin. It was then when the group changed its name to KIPSA and became independent from KAPA. I chose training at KIPSA because I believed that we could move forward by learning from the experience and history of the IPA. I think it was such a meaningful decision of KIPSA to make its decision-making process more democratic rather than authoritative and I also respect the decision was made for the future and not for the immediate benefit. As a candidate representative, I would like to thank KIPSA for laying the groundwork for the organization to develop as what it is now. However, the process of separating KAPA and KPSG was disappointing for me, as I watched some members refusing to accept the non-discrimination policy through democratic process and thereby withdrawing and splitting the group. The news that some analysts even creating new psychoanalyst training programs for psychiatrists only was strange. The information about such programs often would not be wide open and I felt sorry to hear such secret training programs even existed. Sadly, this process has left a painful scar in the history of psychoanalysis in Korea.

Now, I would like to tell you about my training experience. I had been conducting offline psychotherapy with a patient twice a week for several years and decided to convert this to psychoanalysis after consulting with my supervisor. This patient was at first resistant to recognizing the transference, and thus, not only treatment but also the patient's life itself was stalemated for a long time. I proposed the patient get an offline psychoanalysis session four times a week but the patient suggested to make two sessions online owing to the Covid-19 pandemic. The patient's suggestion showed her wish to be special to the therapist. It was hard for me to reject that suggestion due to the influence of projective identification. To initiate a control case, I had to contact the Education Committee and at the time, I was concerned that arguments between the two groups would affect the initiation of my case. My supervisor, the Chair of the Education Committee and my psychoanalyst all had different opinions on non-discrimination policy. Of course, I was aware of the non-involving system. However, in this situation, any candidate would be forced to be in a relatively vulnerable position. I was anxious. The Education Committee did not confirm the case initiation. To initiate the control case, all sessions must be offline and my case did not meet the requirements, which was why it was difficult to get the confirmation as a control case. I explained this to the patient, who was furious with me for weeks after hearing that the suggestion had not been accepted. After the patient expressed her anger toward me, unlike my expectations, there was slight progress in not only the treatment but also in my personal psychoanalysis. I rather came to thank the Education Committee for not permitting the patient's hidden wishes behind the request for two online sessions. Unlike my worries, I could understand better about the fantasy and the interaction between the patient and myself.

I would like to share my expectations and wishes for the candidate training course. What started my psychoanalyst training was a fundamental question about how the human mind works and how it gets better. Of course, there are deeper, more unconscious reasons as well. Maybe it's a global trend but psychiatry in Korea is mostly focused on medication. Unfortunately, the suicide rate in Korea is one of the highest in the world. That is why many Korean candidates feel the need to better understand and have more interest in the human mind. One of the findings I get from my psychoanalytic training is that psychoanalysis, which originated from the Western countries, works well in Korea as well. I came to realize and appreciate the hard work of the senior analysts who tried to incorporate what had been learned in the West to the Korean culture. I am also grateful to the psychoanalysts from the IPA and APsaA for helping us in this regard.

In order for KIPSA and psychoanalysis in Korea to continue to develop, we must be vigilant about the widespread authoritarianism within the Korean culture and maintain the democratic decision-making process as it is now. I believe it is essential to provide candidates an authentic and transparent training environment. Should KIPSA fail to make constant efforts to this end, the invisible wall of authoritarianism between the Institute and candidates will be back in any time. Authoritarianism associated with the Oedipus complex is faintly, yet widely ingrained in the Eastern culture, and it is subtly different from that of the West. It will not be easy for Korea to be completely free from authoritarianism, especially after suffering from the Korean War and military dictatorship in modern times. It is a subject that needs to be dealt within individual analysis but I do think cultural influence exists. I hope KIPSA listens to and opens itself up to candidates, which will facilitate more active interaction between the Institute and candidates than now. I believe such environment will allow candidates to have their own authentic voices as analysts.

I would like to end this letter with some personal notes. The analyst training at KIPSA and my personal analytic experience changed my thought about psychoanalysis and the Institute. I came to realize through the training that how the Institute, which I previously thought was authoritative and one-sided, emphasizes interactive and practical education and my interactions with the patients, analysts, supervisors and the Institute truly helped me grow into a better individual.

During the course of training, I often visited Deoksugung Palace near my office, which is one of the important historical palaces in Korea. Although the palace was built in 1592, it had not been used again until 1897. When the palace was used again, there was a tremendous cultural shift—the Korean government officially began accepting modern western culture. Now, the palace is located harmoniously with skyscrapers in the middle of downtown Seoul. It seems that I wanted to project my mind into this palace and see the harmony between the present and the past. Around that time, I took a picture of Gwangmyeongmun, one of the Palace gates that had not been fully restored yet, wishing to see its complete restoration someday. The gate was removed during the chaotic period of the history and later returned to its rightful place. The gate had been originally connected to the wall and the building, but after returning to its original place, it still has not been restored completely. Just like Gwangmyeongmun, I think it is time the Korean psycho-analytic society settle down again after suffering from all the conflicts and disputes. I hope that KIPSA, which is a provisional society now, will become a component society in near future. I will end this letter by attaching a photo of the above-mentioned Gwangmyeongmun at Deoksugung Palace, hoping it to be fully restored soon.

With warm regards,

— Chang-Jeung Park

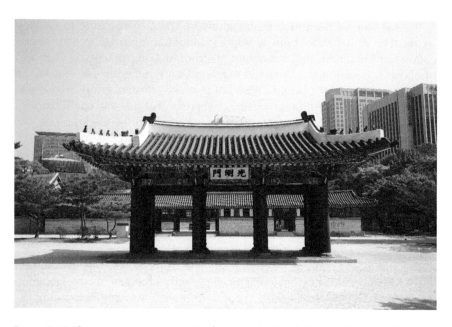

*Figure 34.1* Gwangmyeongmun at Deoksugung in Seoul, Korea. Photograph by the author.

# 35 A letter to the South African Psychoanalytic Association, Johannesburg (2009)

*Zama Radebe and Siobhán Carter-Brown*

*To paint the background of our young institute, The South African Psychoana-lytic Association, was founded in 2009 and offers the first and only psycho-analytic training in Africa. The South African Psychoanalytic Association was founded on the back of the South African Psychoanalytic Initiative, our larger psychoanalytic psychotherapy organisation. Growing out of a society trauma-tised by apartheid, we must recognise that our institute comprises predomi-nantly of white members and candidates. We are two similar aged, female candidates of different race groups. We were part of the second cohort to train in Johannesburg and in that, the first cohort of mixed races. Our institute is small with significant lengths undertaken to have the required number of local training analysts to support an analytic training. A small society means there are continual boundary engagements to navigate. As colleagues in the same cohort, we had separate training analysts but we each then shared our own analysts as our first supervisors with the other. We had our analysts teach us theory and whilst our individual analysis was non reporting, the society is small and the contamination of reality into fantasy is a constant element of training. We feel this is important to emphasise as we fully appreciate the complexity this adds to every layer of engagement. Despite complexities we regret that we didn't play more with the collective encounters and that it was not better facilitated in our training. By collective encounters we mean as colleagues, inside our cohort, with the candidates that trained above us and our Training Committee. This is not divorced from our South African context where othering and racial alienation is prolific.*

—

Dear South African Psychoanalytic Association,

We have crossed over that much anticipated line and are recently graduated as psychoanalysts. It is a great relief that can also feel rather daunting. We are however sustained in the hard-earned knowledge that we are not alone.

DOI: 10.4324/9781003465409-35

The journey to train as psychoanalysts has been an intensely personal endeavour and a journey of immense growth for us both. We however both sit with a regret that making use of the collective was hard for us as candidates. Now that we are through it, we postulate what we can glean from our specific experience for the benefit of our institute and the future candidates we hope will join us. If we wish to consider what might be applicable to our societal dynamics in general, we have to acknowledge the specific dynamics we brought to the table. We were fond of each other from the beginning of our training, but we battled to reach out and pull each other close as friends. Both of us had to navigate a wish to graduate that resulted in us being told that we needed to give it more time. It was painful to get such feedback and made us both worry about whether we would ever grasp this analytic work. Taking the extra time to graduate as well as us committing to reflect on our training together has us contemplating our starting points in training and how that weaves into the collective experience.

One of the reasons Zama trained was that although she had a PhD and was holding a senior position at one of our largest public hospitals, she was lost. She sought psychoanalysis as "I felt that I had disappeared as a person, and I was scared I would not be found. Deadness comes to mind. A tree filled with termites inside. My CV read 'as if', someone else, and there was a lack of connection between who I felt I was and who I read as on paper. It felt like it started as a game where we had been playing hide and seek but I had hidden so much that those who were looking for me had given up on trying to find me. It felt as if I could hear or see the search for me but this was also met with rigidity on my part and ambivalence, wanting to be found but also stuck in the hiding and fearing to be found at the same time." We acknowledge that Zama had her own difficulty with taking up a voice in seminars, but it became a dynamic of the group in general.

Siobhán had seemingly stumbled into psychoanalysis when her supervisor suggested she should train, and she anticipated it would be the ultimate cure for all mental illness. As a parentified child, this was the conscious conduit that led to an analytic encounter where "I was seen as a patient and in pain. Much to my surprise, although I thought I was an open book, I fought it tooth and nail. My analyst stayed firm and slowly over time I let her come close enough for us to dare to see more of me, and for healing to bind the torturous and destructive part of my psyche that had permeated my life in such insidious ways. My strategy to survive had been to be the willing, effective designated leader. It kept me inside, but it also kept people out." The repetition compulsion is indeed strong and in the rupture of losing our group rep, it was then that Siobhán took up the group rep role. Did we somehow then present as coping too well, as a parentified child would, enabling our institute to not fully pick up that we were fumbling?

With hindsight, holding back on graduating was a valuable space, in that, we started to lean into a collegial friendship and share together what we were struggling with. We began to meet socially and embarrassingly uncovered aspects of our histories we had curiously never shared; where we were raised, where we went to school, what our parents were like. Zama did not know that Siobhán was not raised in South Africa until late into the training and so all along had assumed she must know about whiteness in South Africa. Conversely, Siobhán was doing work in a race group and becoming more aware of how pervasive and silencing whiteness could be. She wanted to ask Zama but she was scared that this was her need and that Zama just wanted to be a candidate and not the black candidate. This holding back was not just between us as colleagues, it was how we all seemed to relate as a cohort. Together but somehow on our own. We got to a point where we stopped responding to each other on important messages and we even dropped a seminar with one of the training analysts. We'd like to think we are so special it was just about us, but we trust you have taught us enough to know this must also be an underpinning of dynamics applicable to all training groups.

Despite our formal Clinical Psychology training and many years of further enrichment in the psychodynamic societies of Johannesburg, neither of us had a firm understanding of psychoanalysis before commencing the training. Entering the training we felt like we were the inexperienced, freshly picked candidates. In contrast, the cohort above us seemingly comprised of senior practitioners with vast experience as psychoanalytic psychotherapists, that had dedicated their lives to steeping themselves in the field. It felt like you were not prepared for our lack of understanding as to what psychoanalysis is and how it differs from psychotherapy or psychology. Other than the experience of our own individual analysis, we did not hear an analytic case being presented until we had already taken on our first training cases. We would frequently be told that we were stuck as psychotherapists, but we had little reference as to what psychoanalysis was. In the same breath, the cohort above us seemed to have strong opinions about the direction the training should take, they appeared to be pushing back to the Training Committee about how they felt their training had been lacking, at times it felt like we were out at sea left to swim without a raft.

Our cohort started as a reasonably good number of eight. Initially we recall the feeling of warmth and excitement about being the second cohort in Johannesburg, it felt full of possibilities. It felt like a bubble, like entering a cloud and maybe even blocking out the real world in some instances. A bubble that, when reality intruded, like it always does, we did not grapple with as a group. You will recall that we lost three cohort members in six months before our first year of training was complete. We know the reasons were personal and various. Parts were confusing and unexplained, we traversed extremely tragic circumstances as well as quite the opposite of joy, life and childbirth. Something was not holding. Looking back, it was a huge rupture that we are sure had significant psychic meaning for the group. It was hardly acknowledged either inside the formal training or outside in our informal conversations. We adopted a pressure to turn inwards and to keep pushing despite life around us.

Whilst traversing these losses and still in our first year of training it was decided that the more senior candidates from cohort 1 could attend our lectures with us. We were fragile, just playing with finding our voices and looking back, we shut down, perhaps even spitting out the food that was generously offered. We were all accomplished and ambitious candidates, we all related well individually, yet as a collective, resistance had set in. We wish it had at least felt like an us versus them in the seminar room. If we had banded together and pushed back at the senior candidates or had gotten angry with you, the training committee and our analysts, that split might have been more robust and protective. Instead, it felt more in pieces, diffuse and paranoid inducing. We stopped speaking up about the readings and having comments in the seminars, we let the senior candidates do the work and we grew ever more silent. Often, we seemed to succumb to the position of being infantilised. In many instances we got tied in knots as we scripted feedback to you, anxious about how we would be seen and evaluated.

For both of us we too quickly retreated to giving the authority to the parent. Even though we both had awareness that the senior class joining us for seminars was incredibly uncomfortable we did not dare say it. In our minds you must have thought it through. We felt selfish and could not express the infantile wish; we did not want to share. We felt threatened by their presence and our curiosity and questions could seem too behind and too slow. There was no longer a space to be slow. Then we were asked to evaluate our analysts' teaching. We resisted the format of feedback, and it was met with authoritarian scolding. There was no space to unpack why we were being defiant. We remember a deep insecurity that we did not know enough to critically evaluate our teachers. It fed the retreat to the child-like state and a stronger super-ego relating to the training. There was too much pressure to appear as the good students and that resulted in us not showing what is truly inside.

Of course, all was not lost. Interestingly, we seemed to take an element of connecting outside of our seminar room. We fondly recall a collective space in the playground of Ububele. Only two of the now five members smoked but we would all head out 'to smoke', it was our safe space. There was something comforting about this time in the garden where we would talk and catch up. Retrospectively we wonder why we internalised such a strong punitive super-ego way of relating to our institute and felt we could not be more vulnerable in the seminar room, in the presence of our training analysts. Did the unspoken, unprocessed cleaving of our fellow colleagues leave us with a paranoia as to how we would be expelled? As with all societies, splits happen, and conflict ensues. There were painful institute matters we could not be fully privy to but which directly and significantly affected us both, more often than not we feel we were left on our own with that.

Zama is not the first analyst of colour for the South African Psychoanalytic Association, but as was said in her graduation announcement, "This is a significant milestone in Zama's professional development and also in the history of the South African Psychoanalytic Association and the IPA, as we think Zama might well be the first Zulu speaking psychoanalyst ever!''. The pressure and excitement to have an African speaking, homegrown, black analyst was palpable, but the pressure and expectations embedded in that rarely spoken about. Encompassing two, young black candidates, outwardly we could be seen to be realising the fantasised rainbow nation but unlike the work being done in the South African Psychoanalytic Initiative, it could at times feel like the South African Psychoanalytic Association did not have the desire to enquire about the particular struggles of black candidates. In fairness maybe it was more about capacity, but it is too serious a dynamic for us to foreclose. Similarly with sexual orientation, we were reading homophobic and racist text, yes written in another time and age, but when we raised how difficult it was to read, we were told to ignore that and understand the period from whence it came. We know the South African Psychoanalytic Association offers good enough food, but in highly charged states it is easy to unconsciously foster a paranoia as to whether our institute could really take us in being inexperienced, black or homosexual.

Zama reflects that as a black trainee, I had brought with me a sense of community as well as my own individual experience of how I held the historical context that informed being in class with my white colleagues. It was only later in the training that issues of race were introduced. For some time, it felt like we operated as if these did not apply to us. Racism was out there. I took offence with classes being scheduled on commemorative holidays that signify the remembrance of my history and pain as a black person in South Africa. To this day, I don't feel this was ever fully heard. Being in such an intimate space with my white colleagues felt like such a potentially valuable process with opportunities to engage that I regret that it was somehow lost. Perhaps it was a fear of our hatred that kept our visceral selves out in an attempt to protect but in doing so we deprived ourselves of the opportunity to work from there and find our way to intimacy and closeness. Even if it was a projection and individual dynamics that were primarily at play, not normalising curiosity sets up a dynamic that hinders its very existence. We restricted our ability to play with our differences and inner truths.

We are relatively young and new to learning psychoanalysis, but we are experienced in life and South Africa and we wish to engage in cultivating an understanding and applicability for psychoanalysis in Africa. We need to work in the collective to ascertain what role psychoanalysis plays in feeding the mental health of our starving nation. Can we discuss and bear that in reality some patients get one brief session and are the psychoanalytic theories universal and applicable to our setting? How do we guard against importing psychoanalysis as a privileged, Eurocentric ideology that may repeat and cultivate further splits and alienations in our society. Despite this critique, we have had a rich experience of psychoanalysis in action and can we use the listening and openness that is so particular and rich in psychoanalytic enquiry to really hear and learn from the unique South African psyches and make a difference in spaces that can ripple to further healing.

In essence we wish to advocate for space for primary process. Can we create safe spaces in the training where not only individual analysis, but also the cohort can hold some of the psychic growth that we undergo in this incredible journey. Silencing parts of us, the more disturbed, less put together elements can feel like racism, it was something out there. Exploring fantasy was for our patients to do or for us to take to our analysis. We would love to have had more space for primary processes encouraged during class. It feels like it took us too long to remember we are authorities in our own right and that we had something valuable to say even if we were not qualified.

In closing we hope that our sharing contributes towards more curious and robust engagements at all levels in our collective. We also hope that we can be part of cultivating an institute that holds space for the candidates and its members to be messy and uncertain, to play with ideas and to dare to explore the stupid. Safety and trust need to be cultivated and protected especially in the face of mixed race and diversity. We believe psychoanalysis can play a vital role in the healing of South Africa but has to do so humbly and with a desire to listen to the South African unconscious, using the power of free association and analytic listening that simultaneously guards against imposing a Eurocentric, individual theory on the African mind.

— Zama Radebe & Siobhán Carter-Brown

# 36 A letter to the Estonian-Latvian Psychoanalytic Society, Tallin and Riga (2010)

*Rolands Ivanovs*

*My psychoanalytical home is the Estonian-Latvian Psychoanalytic Society (ELPS) which is a Provisional Society of the International Psychoanalytical Association (IPA). Training process of the ELPS is organised according to Eitingon model. Basic requirements for graduation are*

- *Four years of theoretical training (two weekends per month)*
- *Two cases under supervision*
- *The completion of personal training analysis*

*The Estonian-Latvian Psychoanalytic society is a very young and developing group which was founded in 2010 and comprises colleagues from two neighbouring Baltic countries—Latvia and Estonia. Shared historical longings and aspirations for independence from totalitarian realm and oppression brought us together as close relatives and laid the foundations for psychoanalysis in our countries. Some important socio-political events illustrate this common thriving for freedom:*

- *The Baltic Way was a peaceful political demonstration which took place on 23 August 1989 when approximately two million people joined their hands forming a 600 km long human chain through the Baltic countries, thus demonstrating their unity in efforts towards freedom from the Soviet Union and commemoration of the 50th anniversary of the Molotov-Ribbentrop Pact*
- *Lithuania, Estonia and Latvia declared the reestablishment of their independence from the Soviet Union in the spring of 1990 and had to defend it with non-violent resistance barricades of January 1991 which culminated in bloody incidents when declarations were pronounced illegal by the USSR's central authority*
- *After a failed coup in Moscow, the Soviet Government finally recognised the independence of all three Baltic States on 6 September 1991*

DOI: 10.4324/9781003465409-36

*It was a new beginning poignantly reflected in the lines of the Hymn for The Baltic Way* "The Baltics Are Waking Up!" (1989):

*"And the sea starts to wave,*
*Three sisters wake up from the sleep,*
*Come to stand for themselves.*
*The Baltics are waking up, The Baltics are waking up,*
*Lithuania, Latvia, Estonia!"*

*The Baltic Republics were the first in the former Soviet Union to conduct democratic elections and to declare their independence. Withdrawal of Russian troops from all Baltic States followed some years later and was completed only in August 1994. Skrunda-1, The last Russian military radar in the Baltics, officially suspended operations in August 1998. We were lucky! Our historical struggles created a strong emotional bond with the Ukrainian people who are now fighting for their independence and freedom. We feel their pain and admire their courage and fighting spirit!*

*A very interesting and not widely known fact is that our peaceful "divorce" from the former Soviet Union and development of "new" Baltic large-group identities was facilitated by a psychoanalyst. Members of the University of Virginia's Center for the Study of Mind and Human Interaction (CSMHI) under the guidance of psychoanalyst Vamik Volkan created a multidisciplinary team that brought together representatives of opposing large groups for dialogues in all three Baltic States from 1992 to 1996 holding fast to a most significant technical psychoanalytic principle: the facilitating team—members of CSMHI—had no formulas for solving the Baltic Republics' problems; each country would find its own solutions (Volkan, 2013). It was a time of* **awakening** *and* **freedom** *for the Baltic States. It was a time for psychoanalysis! The fall of Iron Curtain opened the doors for psychoanalysis in Latvia and Estonia.*

**Latvian Association for Psychodynamic Psychiatry, Psychosomatic Medicine and Psychotherapy (LPTA) was** *founded in 1991 almost immediately after regaining of independence as part of the Latvian Medical Society. The First World Congress of Latvian Doctors in 1989, which became one of the most important events of the Third National Awakening,[1] facilitated the reestablishment of lost bonds between colleagues from all over the world (O'Connor, 2003). Teachers from Western Europe and Canada started to visit Latvia. First group of 24 Latvian psychotherapists were enrolled in a three-year psychodynamic psychotherapy training organised in Eskilstuna, Sweden from 1992 to 1995. Estonian colleagues went to study to Finland. Connection of Latvian and Estonian psychotherapists grew stronger when some Estonian colleagues became training therapists for Latvian colleagues in training. In 1994 Department of Psychosomatic medicine and psychotherapy was established at the Riga Stradins University and began to deliver educational courses in psychotherapy for medical students. These were different kind of seminars which contrasted very much with didactic training in human anatomy, physiology* and biochemistry. Teachers were much younger, more passionate and more interested in our thoughts, feelings and our personalities. I still remember how we read Freud's case of Little Hans together in one of the seminars. Encouraged by these enthusiastic teachers I started to attend the meetings of LPTA, which were very inspiring and well-attended at that time. **Awakening** was in the air! What was very important that these meetings were open for everybody who was interested in psychotherapy and who had a courage to attend these meetings. Even a special status of a Contributing Member was created for those who were not members but were interested and supported development of psychotherapy in Latvia. I felt very personally connected to this movement because one of the first psychotherapy residents became my therapist. I was also awakened from my own anxieties, conflicts and melancholic feelings. It was a powerful experience, it was experience of love. In one of these meetings I have heard for the first time about Psychoanalytical Summer Schools organised by the Han Groen-Prakken Psychoanalytic Institute for Eastern Europe (PIEE). It sounded so mysterious and enticing, giving way to a lot of fantasies. But my destined Summer School was yet to come. Recently I have learned to know that idea of Psychoanalytical Summer Schools was born in Estonia and in funny circumstances. One of the PIEE meetings took place in Laulasmaa, a small Estonian resort village, in a wintertime at a Soviet time "SPA" hotel left without heating. Participants had to improvise to stay warm, including a lot of dancing. Thereafter Estonian psychoanalyst Endel Talvik proposed the idea about Psychoanalytical Summer Schools which was accepted as a very justified and brilliant idea. Nevertheless, tradition of dancing remained alive also in Summer Schools. It turned out that the Han Groen-Prakken PPIEE was the Institute where most of our teachers received their psychoanalytic training. It was a joint creation of the IPA and the European Psychoanalytical Federation (EPF) to **lay foundation for psychoanalysis in post-communist countries where** psychoanalysis was largely forbidden until 1989. The PIEE gathered experienced analysts from all over the world, including Aira Laine, Paolo Fonda, Antonius Stufkens, John Kafka, Gabor Szönyi, Gary Goldsmith, Abigail Golomb, Gilbert Diatkine, Michel Vincant, Patricia Daniel, Haydee Faimberg, Patrick Casement and many others. Some of teachers had personal historical connection with Eastern Europe. Encouraged and inspired by doctor Arkadijs Pancs who was the pioneering psychoanalyst in Latvia I finally ventured to my first PIEE Summer schools in 2005 and 2006. It was a unique and unforgettable experience, because you could feel the warmth, wisdom, interest in your thoughts and feelings. You could feel the care and love of teachers for psychoanalysis and their patients. And very importantly—you could share the tradition of dancing and celebrating life together! Such an experience cannot leave you indifferent and makes you want to get closer and belong to this family. That's how Summer Schools fuelled my wish for **belonging** to psychoanalytic community that, as a powerful current, carried me to the banks of the ELPS. Training process at ELPS, according to an IPA compliant training programme, was first started on 2013. And five years later the second group

*of trainees which consisted of six Estonian and four Latvian candidates includ-
ing me was launched into an infinite universe of psychoanalysis.*

Dear Institute and dear colleagues, the key words that come to my mind
when I am thinking about my psychoanalytical journey and history of ELPS
are **gratitude, love, freedom, awakening** and **belonging.**

At first, I want to express my deep **gratitude** for accepting me to your psychoanalytic family, creating and giving me home to a professional identity formation. Reading Fred Busch's book *Dear Candidate* I have realised how many
obstacles and difficulties analysts of previous generations had to face in their
psychoanalytical journeys. Each generation had its own historical context and
challenges. Our teachers had to travel abroad for personal shuttle analysis
and training or even had to move for some time to another country. Now we
can enjoy the luxury of being trained in our homelands. I am so proud of our
teacher's enthusiasm, courage and perseverance to build our psychoanalytical home. I think it is a good example of binding force that oversteps borders
of countries, nationality and language. What matters is **love** and passion for
psychoanalysis. It feels like a solid, good and nourishing foundation.

Dear Institute, I think that term "universe" captures the infinity of psychoanalytic education much better than "training programme". It was exciting
and at the same time very frustrating to dive into the ocean of psychoanalytic
literature and to realise that you will never be able to read everything that is
written until now. I would have liked to have received a containment for this
greedy fantasy and anxiety much earlier in my training.

It was a very enriching and mind opening experience to have a home
in two countries at the same time and to study with Latvian and Estonian
colleagues with so diverse and interesting backgrounds. Respectful, lov-
ing, accepting and supporting attitude in our group cured me from the split
between doctors and psychologists working in psychotherapy field which had
deep roots in Latvia. The main training language was English but it was not
possible to avoid Estonian, Latvian, Russian and even a bit of German. During
the process of training I feel that some part of me has converted into Estonian.
Our training was organised with weekend seminars once in two weeks con-
secutively in Riga and then in Tallinn. It included regular traveling which gave
a possibility to spend more time together and get closer to each other. I guess
this created a closer emotional and historical bond with our teachers who had
to travel a lot in their training process and we continued this tradition. Each
teacher had his/her own style of conducting seminars. Similar to the relationship between parents and children we had to adapt to each other. Dear
institute, for me the most challenging were seminars without any guidance
from the side of a teacher. Sometimes it felt like an abandonment in a helpless state and fear to waste useful body of knowledge conveyed in articles. It
took some time until we managed to use this space creatively. I guess it would
have been less frustrating if teachers had explained the rationale behind their
way of conducting seminars from the very beginning.

Dear Institute, it was a great idea to organise separate meetings for new candidates and candidates of previous group to share their experiences and discuss ways of dealing with difficulties in the study process. Unfortunately, such meetings were too rare. I would have liked to see them at every meeting of the Society. I think it would strengthen the links between the different generations and within our group as a whole, as well as bridging the gap between candidates and analysts.

The most difficult time was spring of 2020 when COVID crisis caught us off guard. Travel and meeting restrictions shook our usual training process. There was confusion and uncertainty in everyone. After some interruption and hesitation, we continued training remotely in Zoom. For some of my colleagues this pause felt too long, for some it was an unexpected opportunity to take a brake from intensive training process. We seem to have adapted well to it, although it could not replace the warmth and liveliness of the face-to-face meetings. The COVID crisis revealed a split in our teachers of how to continue. Some teachers considered that it is very essential to continue training in person not to lose the interpersonal quality of psychoanalytical education, some teachers considered remote training as a question of personal choice. It felt like a quarrel between parents. It seems that COVID crisis provoked previously unresolved issues in teacher relations. It was very sad and upsetting that some teachers used this situation, seminars and candidates as a battleground to escalate their conflicts. Luckily there was a happy ending! It is reassuring to know that our Society is still under surveillance of an IPA Sponsoring Committee (our symbolical grandparents) which includes Leena Klockars from Finland and Thijs de Wolf from Netherlands who were following the development of ELPS and hopefully supervising our "parents", too. This year with a very warm-hearted Society meeting and participation of our "grandparents" we celebrated completion of our four years long theoretical training programme. Of course, it does not feel as an end but rather a new beginning for me and I am sure that for some of my colleagues, too.

Dear Institute, only writing this letter I realised what a long way I have made and how far I still have to go. That the path to my training was much longer than the formal training itself. That my formation as an analyst started long ago and that there is no way back! Psychoanalysis is where I belong. This is my family that goes beyond my Society, beyond geographical borders and limits of time, that connects me to colleagues around the world and colleagues who are no longer with us. **Psychoanalysis is a love that awakens, a link to infinity!**

Dear Institute, during my training years I have realised that it is up to you how much you receive from your training. Teachers, especially if they are passionate and welcoming, can open the doors but you have to make the necessary steps. It is up to you if you look for additional training options, like mind opening, connecting IPSO, IPA and EPF events. I guess that for me the most unique and vivid experience during my journey were the Psychoanalytical Summer Schools initially organised by the Han Groen-Prakken PIEE and since 2015 taken over by the European Psychoanalytic Institute (EPI). I really admire the work done by the EPI board **Igor M. Kadyrov, Christoph Walker, Endel Talvik and Tomas Kajokas who invested so much energy and time to make it possible. There is something magical when teachers and candidates come together from all over the world in nice, warm, sunny place for one week and immerse themselves in psychoanalytic universe alongside celebrating life. It is surprisingly transformative experience after which you are not the same person anymore!**

**I wish that international psychoanalytical community and my Institute could preserve and continue this unique tradition! You can count on me!**

— Rolands Ivanovs

## Note

1 *The Latvian National Awakening* (Latvian: *latviešu [or latvju] tautas atmoda*) refers to three distinct but ideologically related National revival movements:
The First Awakening refers to the national revival led by Young Latvians from the 1850s to the 1880s culminating in the First All-Latvian Song Festival in Riga in 1873
The Second Awakening or "New Current" was the movement that led to the proclamation of Latvian independence in 1918
The Third Awakening was the movement that led to the restoration of Latvia's independence in the "Singing Revolution" of 1987–1991 (O'Connor, 2003)

# 37 A letter to Societatea Română de Psihanaliză, Bucharest, Romania (2011)

*Carla Pînzaru*

*The founding of the Societatea Română de Psihanaliză (SPR) is an impor-tant moment in the development of psychoanalysis in Romania, which went through three main stages. The first stage, which ended with the establish-ment of communism in Romania (23 August 1944), imposed by the USSR, was characterised by a good and synchronous reception of psychoanalysis, especially in medical circles. As early as 1913, doctoral theses on psychoanal-ysis began to be defended at the Faculty of Medicine in Bucharest. By 1940, 10 such theses had been defended.*

*Romania's communist Academy officially condemned psychoanalysis, which would become one of the favourite targets of ideological attacks. Clinically it became clandestine. During this difficult period they practiced: Constantin Vlad, Ion Popescu-Sibiu, Ion Vianu, Eugen Papadima, Nadia Bujor, Irena Talaban, Horia Bejat, Augustin Cambosie, Radu Clit, Vasile Dem. Zamfirescu, Vera Șandor and others. Some of Eugen Papadima's analyses turned out to be didactic (training).*

*After the collapse of communism at the end of 1989, the third stage of psy-choanalysis in Romania began. Its main goals were: a) psychoanalytic prac-tice ceases to be clandestine; b) legal possibility of professional association (constitution of the Romanian Psychoanalytic Society); c) elimination of ideo-logical prohibitions on psychoanalysis and the possibility to publish without restrictions psychoanalytic literature; d) official recognition of psychoanalysis as a subject of study in higher education; e) permanent contact with Western psychoanalysts.*

*Between 2000–2011, the SRP had the official name of "Romanian Society of Psychoanalysis—Study Group". Following the recognition as direct mem-bers of the IPA, and four of the members of the group (Vera Șandor, Brîndușa Orășanu, Eugen Papadima, Vasile Dem. Zamfirescu) were given the status of psychoanalysts trainers and supervisors.*

DOI: 10.4324/9781003465409-37

*This professional group initiated the Training Program which complies with the IPA criteria and consists of:*

- *personal analysis with an SRP training analyst—minimum 4 years/3–4 times a week, on the couch;*
- *compulsory theoretical seminars—minimum 4 years;*
- *two clinical supervisions of minimum two years each, with two different SRP supervisors.*

*With the IPA Congress in Mexico, August 2011, SRP became a provisional IPA Society.*

—

Dear Institute,

It has been several weeks since I received, with a lot of joy and enthusiasm, an invitation to write you a letter. A rich, continuous and restructuring working through ensued that carried me back in time, seven years ago, when I applied to become an IPA candidate. At that time, I had to write an essay to answer the question "What can you tell us about your interest in psychoanalysis and your wish to become a psychoanalyst?". I wrote then that this question came back to my mind quite frequently during my personal analysis, and I came up with a different answer every time. Today, I would say that for someone who is undergoing the working through of a psychoanalysis, this is not surprising at all. Nevertheless, for me, as I started my analysis for a painful situation I was going through at that moment of my life, and not as a training analysis, the recollection of my answer has a touch of humour as well. One or two years later after the debut of my analysis, I returned to my old interest in psychoanalysis and started studying for my second university degree, in psychology. Why am I taking this detour through the history of my training years? It is because during the last few years—I am now in the middle of my second analysis under supervision, part of my training—another question arose, a question that I have put together clearly only with the occasion of this invitation to write to you about "what it means to be a psychoanalyst".

This might seem hilarious at first—how can anyone not know what a psychoanalyst is, but to be in the middle of a training she chose exactly because she wanted to become a psychoanalyst. Actually, my intuition tells me this is a question the answer of which places us face to face with ourselves from the moment we first wish for something and until the end of our lives, continuously and in a different way every time. Once we started off on this route, somewhere deep down in our hearts we know there is no turning back, we cannot "part ways" with psychoanalysis, not even when we tend to abandon it.

When I started the training process, after having already undergone quite a few years of personal analysis, I had no idea I had not gone through its hardest part of all. I had been undergoing my personal analysis before the beginning of training. Well, for me that was the anchor allowing me to be able to cope with the *transference,* in its several different shapes it took later on, when relationships became more complicated, when my analyst, my supervisors and my colleagues got closer and closer.

I stepped into the institute with a lot of curiosity. I was looking for a better family, a more empathetic one, an ideal one even—another commonplace for senior psychoanalysts, who I think are pretty used to their candidates' phantasms. I was hoping to learn many things, to understand psychoanalysis from those ones who had been practising it successfully and, at the same time, I was afraid I did not know the language they would use to talk to us, the candidates. This was a fear feeding from the fact that over there, in Romania, all candidates study together during the *theoretic—clinical seminars,* regardless of their year of training. How would I be able to comprehend a paper at the level that another colleague would do, one who had been studying psychoanalysis for four years? One who maybe has already undergone an individual supervision?

My first big surprise was to see how different the lecturers were from what I was expecting, how *differently* they "understood" psychoanalysis. Instead of feeling at peace, my restlessness increased. For me, there was just one single psychoanalysis. I was looking sometimes at the lecturers, sometimes at my colleagues, trying to see whether I was the only one who felt this way and that maybe my personal lens was distorted. It was my curiosity that saved me, because I decided to try to understand the language of each and every one of them, as I was convinced that, if they are there, the trainers also have a *mutual language* that evaded me.

Shortly afterwards, I received an email from the president of the Training Committee with an announcement about a colloquium in Budapest. I cannot remember the main topic exactly, but it was about legacy and the history of psychoanalysis in Hungary. Not accidentally, as a teenager, my first encounter with Freud's lectures was connected to the concept of the *unconscious.* It reverberated into my numerous questions regarding my family of origin that I had not understood yet, but that I had been striving to ever since I was a little girl. I was to go to Budapest on my own and, picking up on one of my colleague's idea, to talk to the people from IPSO and find out how we could join the organisation. I did not know much about IPSO as an organisation and did not know one single colleague outside Romania. I was in my first training year.

All emotions included, I had a series of meetings the results of which I still carry with me today. I came back, we got together and, years later, we are still a group, which is part of IPSO and participates at its events.

However, the Budapest colloquium had meant a lot more. The history of psychoanalysis in Hungary is impressive, touching and the fact that, in such a brave way, both psychoanalysts and candidates were able to speak freely about the difficulties they had encountered in the society over time gave me a lot of hope. Especially when Hungary is Romania's neighbour country. My grandfather on my mother's side was Hungarian-only now, when I am writing to you, do I have this revelation I do not remember having before.

I returned to Romania and, in a way, I felt I could relax. There are *different perspectives* on psychoanalysis everywhere inside institutions. That was for me, at best, a first minuscule psychical integration. (I have to mention here that my analysis was closer to the classical theory, so the term *conflict* was familiar to me in this way, too.)

I had been working with patients, as a psychotherapist with a previous training in psychoanalytical psychotherapy, but not for a long time. I was a rookie on all fronts, as they say. So, my second encounter with reality came up shortly afterwards: the lack of affiliation. There was this idea going around that we were not part of the society, as we were not psychoanalysts and that the group of candidates had to take care of themselves. We used to meet the lecturers only when attending their seminars and, twice a year, during the summer school and the conference the Society was organising. We were utterly confused. We had just been to Paris, participating in another event organised by IPSO at SPP,[1] where we found a beautiful headquarters, several conference rooms, a library where we could buy books and magazines that we would have otherwise found only in antiquarian bookshops. However, more than anything else, we had learnt for the first time that a candidate of this society could get patients for psychoanalysis from a senior who consults the patient and send him for a personal analysis to a candidate in training. This made quite an impression on me, but, just like anyone else coming from the Eastern Bloc, I accepted, with a sign of resignation that we are not in the same place as France. But there is hope, isn't there? If it hadn't been any, how else could we work with the people's suffering, with the construction and deconstruction; how else could we hope a man would find his/her resources to build something better for himself/herself?

I decided right then and there that, as a representative of the Romanian candidates, I would make sure we were a united group. The first step towards affiliation is existence itself. It was then when I had my first meeting with two of the representatives of the Society, in our little room in a chic Bucharest neighbourhood. The mere fact that the Society and the Institute started getting a face, a voice, was comforting. This is a detail that maybe you, from inside these institutions, cannot sense anymore. As long as we could talk to each other, it meant we existed, that we were acknowledging each other's existence.

The words above make me think about the continuous working through of the analyst-analysand dyad. Together we are jumping into waters, most of the times murky, unknown waters, swimming in uncertainties; however, at the beginning and at the end of the session we look each other in the eye and know we are both alive, distinct human beings, with our own existence outside the sessions.

There is a third aspect I have experienced, and it refers to *atmosphere*. Our group seemed to lack vitality. I was always asking myself whether I should look for the answer strictly inside our group or whether it was something more than that. Something like a devitalisation, one present in the entire institution. If this was the case, what was causing it? Surely, I could not have answered this question on my own, no matter how much effort I would have put into it. So, I relied on IPSO again and continued to take part in their activities, meet colleagues from other countries and talk freely with each other about the experiences in our countries. At the same time, I was excited our Romanian group included colleagues who found inspiration in my encouragement and that is how we started—and continue—to organise intervision groups, where we can discuss clinical cases and anything else that concerns us. Every now and then, we have meetings that really make our lives easier, as we discover we have similar questions, worries or frustrations. We haven't reached that point where we would have that high level of openness and trust allowing us to share our concerns with the Institute. Sometimes I think it is detrimental to us for these concerns to reach only personal analysts and that we are never able to share them in reality with the ones who can listen to them and address them in reality as well. I am still preoccupied with the influence the communist society has had over us, over future generations, though I refuse to look only through the victim's lens. I was 14 at the moment of Ceaușescu's exit and the fall of communism. As a kid, my memories are rather nice, but as an adult, I feel my generation too carries the print of that regime. It is difficult for us to have a voice, we are afraid to speak freely, we fear the judgement of others and especially, we fear being rejected. On the other side, people easily tend to go towards power, authority, wait for obedience. The history of the past few years has shown us that most of the institutions in Romania fail their missions because of that. Nevertheless, psychoanalysts have the advantage of being capable to see this whole picture more easily and, thanks to psychoanalysis, this includes the moment when they themselves are part of it. Unfortunately, communism taught us that evil is always outside of us, that it lies in the other one and never in us. Moreover, those who have been "possessed" by this evil ended up in prisons, tortured, or were exiled or uprooted. It is surprising that psychoanalysis or psychoanalytic psychotherapy, as clandestine the attempt to practice them as it was, have survived those dreadful times in Romania.

That feeling of lack of vitality within the group has sometimes been associated with the lack of interest. However, the mistrust, the helplessness, the confusion, the lack of hope, the depression, all of that can devitalise a human being, a group of people, an institution.

Later on, around the middle part of my training, I felt something was changing. Something was changing in me, but also outside of me. Curiosity, in its best sense, that stayed unaltered and the wish to know more things were the two values I relied on. Slowly but surely, I started to feel more at ease asking questions, speaking more openly during our working meetings with the lecturers, discovering sources in each paper studied and in the seniors' explanations for the new connections my mind was making. The fact that I was already working with patients, and at the same time, I was continuing my analysis helped me a lot. I had already had my first supervision done, part of my training, but had already had the experience of three previous supervisions to become psychotherapist. I also chose foreign supervisors, from Israel and France, thus making sure my experiences were as diverse as possible. I could say I felt safe during this experience. We had created more space for dialogue, and I do not think it was due only to the formulation of transference, though this played an important part in it, but also to the reality in which both the candidates and our trainers participated. I felt we had become more excited to share, even if we, the candidates, did not have the experience of a psychoanalyst. This relief that I felt reassured me that personal analysis is the pillar of the training of a psychoanalyst. Without it, I believe transference is just a concept. I remember a professor from the university, a psychotherapist of a different school of psychotherapy. He tried to describe transference during one of his lectures (unfortunately, while trying to denigrate psychoanalysis, I must say). That was so difficult for him that in the end, the conclusion was that the patient confuses the analyst with his parent. In this case, I wonder, how could we deeply comprehend what the unconscious is? I was outraged, but then I was not able to find the right words or the courage to confront him. My only certainty was the injustice done to psychoanalysis.

Once I sat down in the armchair behind the couch, everything seemed different somehow. It was just as if I was having an analysis or an accelerated analysis done, without realising it. If, at the beginning, I was literally afraid, sometimes I felt paralysed by what I was feeling when I was interacting with my patients, gradually, I started to be able to think. Then, around two years later, I was under the impression I heard my analyst talking through my words or through the tones of my voice. It struck me and allowed me to shake it off and ask myself whether I am authentic or not and, if not, when exactly this happened. After a while, I listened to Cristopher Bollas speaking in Paris for us, the candidates, saying (I approximately quote) it would take us five years to forget everything we know from our analyst and supervisors and to be ourselves in our practice. From this point on, more and more breakthroughs ensued, closely connected to our own going through and, gradually I was less afraid of the *countertransference,* so that I was able to pay attention to it. I was still undergoing my personal analysis, so I was astonished to see I was working on several layers at the same time when I am in my practice with my patients. I believe this was the moment when the question "What does it mean to be a psychoanalyst?" started to take shape. I was not regarding training as a journey in stages, its final purpose being the assessment for becoming an IPA member. It had become more and more obvious to me that I had to become a psychoanalyst on the inside or, even more, to discover whether there was a psychoanalyst taking shape inside myself. All the transformations I was going through were leading me to the conclusion that *becoming a psychoanalyst is a process in itself,* same as elaboration in personal analysis. That encompasses numerous loops, comebacks, stagnations, revelations and then loops again. At the end of all these, one can simply feel the transformation, but retrospectively. This is pretty much how I was imagining this training. In a way, it never stops. Perhaps *psychoanalyst* is a title, a profession, a term for a method one uses in his/her work, but this has nothing to do with being a psychoanalyst per se. I do not know how to put this, but today, when I am writing these lines, I believe it is important one *feels like a psychoanalyst* first and foremost. As in this field of activity you cannot work without being honest, each one of us will have the intuition of the moment when we are ready for the assessment, regardless of its outcome.

Dear Institute, I will talk to you about the part that proved rather difficult for me, as I did not understand it: the politics of an organisation. I have always imagined that, were there a more open dialogue between the institute and its candidates, reality would be clearer, more intelligible. After all, the transferences over the institution, a lecturer, a supervisor, etc. are inevitable, impossible to control and the only place where they can be worked on is between the analyst and the analysand or, later on, in self-analysis. Why am I writing this? We talk—more or less explicitly—about these transferences, in theory, as if they would make a more open institutional relationship between trainers and candidates impossible. However, I wonder whether an ambiguous reality, one we cannot talk about at all, but all of us are aware of, results in even more nuisance than transference does. Perhaps these words I am writing now are something new for you. Perhaps you are not even aware there are thoughts like that in the candidates' world. That is precisely why I am sharing them with you. It helps us to know that even if we do not belong to the Society, we are part of the Institute. It helps us to know any contribution we bring to the Society, be it in the scientific or administrative activity, is appreciated, even if we are simply candidates. It helps us to know it is not a shame to say out loud when we do not understand a concept and to know you have the patience to help us discover it. After all, it helps us to know your trainers as well, dear Institute, were once candidates and experienced similar feelings. And, considering the Romanian Psychoanalytical Society is relatively young and maybe not all its trainers had a candidate status when it was founded, it helps us to know you can regard those who took this journey with understanding.

I would personally like to feel the joy of being a psychoanalyst that your members feel, dear Institute and for that joy to be shared with us. We are now aware of the fact that you are there, that we are here and we are still waiting to be together with you, just like this has recently seemed to start being possible . . .

Feeling grateful for everything we have lived through together, but also hopeful for a near, more clear future,

— Carla Pînzaru

## Note

1  Société Psychanalytique de Paris.

# 38 A letter to the Taiwan Center for the Development of Psychoanalysis, Taipei (2018)

*Nancy Pei-Ling Yu*

*In 2014, Taiwan Center for the Development of Psychoanalysis was established by a group of psychoanalytic-oriented clinicians, with the goal of forming a psychoanalytic community and hopefully becoming an IPA component society to conduct local training. It was formally recognized as Allied Center by IPA in 2006. According to the procedural code of IPA, a new group could develop through the progressive process of Study Group, Provisional Society, and finally component Society. Therefore, forming a Study Group became the next step of Taiwan Center.*

*It takes at least four IPA affiliated analysts to form a study group. In Taiwan, senior colleagues went abroad to pursue their training of psychoanalysts. One by one, they returned from London, Paris, and USA. Some colleagues sought recognition via the route of "direct member", as they have received an equivalent mode of training. The group finally reached its first step of success in 2015, thus came Taiwan Study Group. Since 2018, with already eight IPA-affiliated analysts and the assistance of IPA sponsoring committee, Taiwan Study group officially launched a training system. One thing particular about us is that analysts were trained in various places, in various "schools" and together constitute a "plurality" of theoretical orientations. Dr. Chia-Chang Liu described it as "Formosa Model"—from geographical and ecological view to the human and societal compositions, Taiwan is characterized by a high level of diversity in terms of people, language, culture, and politics. So does the development of psychoanalysis in this island.*

*I was one of the founding members of Taiwan Center, Secretary General for the first eight years after 2004, and one of the first group of candidates. My "teachers" in the institute are, in a way, friends and colleagues for me.*

—

Dear Institute:

Being one of the first few Taiwan candidates is a unique experience. When I knew that my application for psychoanalytic training was accepted, I feel so happy and proud of myself, and ourselves, too!

DOI: 10.4324/9781003465409-38

I still remember how excited I was when I went to London for my master's degree in 2002, and for the first time I got the chance to meet those "real" psychoanalysts. To me, analysts were like some kind of mysterious gurus, who knew every secret of human minds. At that time, I never imagined that I would have anything to do with psychoanalytical training. When Dr. Jung-Yu Tsai[1] invited me to join Taiwan Center, I thought, well, it sounded nice to continue something related to psychoanalysis. During the process of forming Study Group, even though I also filled-in my application form direct member, I did not really think that it would be something serious! Rather, I was trying to figure out how far the distance between where I was and the goal of being

qualified as an analyst. Honestly, I was still occupied with my daily psychiatric practice, and was not sure if I could live on a private practice of psychotherapist. When, during my direct member interview, Rudi and Michael[2] told me to pursue local training, it was like an announcement: "you can't put your feet on both side of things; either you stay amateur of psychoanalysis, or you make an effort to become a real analyst". Now it is the real game!

I have to confess that the request of filling-in our application form twice (in English and in Mandarin) really annoyed me, and I half-jokingly wrote down: "I am sorry I don't have a more bumpy and interesting personal history to offer". I mean, being a psychiatry and psychanalyst is like a rebellion against my parents' expectation of me. Nevertheless, my experience of having an interview with our sponsoring committee was inspiring. Rudi and Michael[2] asked me a question during the selection interview: how did I see my position in Taiwan Center and my relationship with you, and how was I going to cope with the change of this relationship? It is a bit complicated. For many years, as Secretary General of Taiwan Center, I was like a daughter in the family of administrative team—managing household business and took part in decision making, but not quite among the same rank of you, my senior colleagues. Now as a candidate, I am going back to where I belong to and stay with my siblings. My new identity as a candidate is not only about fulfilling the requests of training, but also about a change of my professional identity from a psychiatrist to a psychoanalyst. I will also begin a different relationship with you, dear institute!

My first challenge would be to find a new analyst. I was left with very limited choices—you were either my friends or my colleagues, we have been so familiar that you are everything but "mysterious gurus", as those British gentlemen and old ladies were. As a result, I chose someone who was more or less unfamiliar yet highly regarded in our professional circle. The fact that she lives in a city 150 kilometers away from where I am is an undeniable burden for me. I started a new routine of traveling back-and-forth between two different cities twice a week, spending time on high-speed train, metro, bus, and Uber. It takes a lot of time, and I doubted if it is worthwhile.

I feel guilty when I secretly compare my new analyst with my previous one in London—I guess the first love was always the best. It was the prototype for me to measure any following experience. I thought doing analysis in my mother tongue would be easier, but it turns out to be a near and far experience. Intellectually I know that personal analysis is more of my personal need than an obligation, and that our analysts will not provide any information or comments in occasions when we candidates are under evaluation; yet in such a small group like us, it is extremely difficult to maintain anonymous in personal analysis. When I complain about my supervisors or seminar teachers in my sessions, I fear that I might provoke splitting or rivalry among you. When I complain about my fellow candidates, I fear that I would either influence your opinions towards them, or you might think it is my problem because you know each of them. I guess it is not about the problem of trust; rather, it is about my fantasy of a big family where each family member has multiple roles and multiple co-existing relationships. I, in every sense as the eldest child, oscillated between the parental and children's generations, and struggled to remain undisturbed.

Eventually it has been a rewarding experience as it enables me to better work through my own oedipal issues. My first analysis was too short! Pandora's box was opened, and I only got a glimpse of the content but soon it was time to leave London. For many years, I kept thinking of picking up my unfinished analysis, but eventually did not put this idea to action. Were it not for the occasion of seeking psychoanalytic training, I probably would still succumb to my resistances. Or, could it be possible that one of the purposes of my training is to finally get back on the couch?

Theoretical study is my favorite part of the training. I like the way our curriculums are organized and taught, although the volume of reading materials is a bit, well, too "generous". I did not force myself to finish them all; after all, we've got our whole life to read them, why hurry? Dear Institute, we are lucky to have teachers from different continents and schools. The contrast and comparison open our mind and eyes. I also like the way you organize our seminars. It is amazing to see how each of you would work differently on the same case material. The scary part is tutoring. I don't know how other institutes manage this problem, but there are only less than ten of you! We cannot attend our own analyst's seminar; therefore, it is both a privilege and a torture to do tutoring. Imagine a one-on-one or one-on-two home tutor who force you to read through a whole bunch of articles! No exaggeration, because our tutors have read all of them too! Dear Institute, I appreciate the great effort of you to spend every Saturday afternoon on assisting new generation of future analysts to learn, to think, and to work. Of course, it's not without chaos or pain. You are new in this training program, too! Some of you keep revising your reading lists, renewing your ways of teaching, and (not that secretly) arguing among you about ways to improve this whole training process. I remember at one moment we were requested to give feedback to our teachers, of course anonymously. Candidates faced the dilemma of communicating freely or creating tension between teachers and students. The avoidance of conflicts with authority is both cultural and projection of our own phantasies. Some of us became paranoid about being evaluated and criticized, and it took us some time to finally feel safe enough. When we feel safe enough, we may finally say to ourselves that it is alright if we are far from being perfect; we could learn to be better together.

What follows is the most difficult part of training: finishing our control cases. As supervisors play a decisive role in selecting the timing of requesting for permission of a control case, but it is Training Committee who holds the power of making final decisions, we are again confronted with a lot of anxiety and projection. Unlike the atmosphere of learning didactics as a group, we candidates have to face anxiety and frustration alone. Even though my supervisors are very supportive, I still find it very difficult. One of the reasons might be that we are all under evaluation. Our sponsoring committee are supposed to offer help to the whole institute to run a solid training program, just like analysts are supposed to help candidate to learn. It is inevitable that we become defensive from time to time, when we feel that the institute is in the position of an adolescent. We are allowed to function independently, but only to the extent that our sponsoring committee thinks we are capable of. On one hand, according to my experience of contacting Rudi and Michael, I trust they are always there to support us; on the other hand, I feel that if I fail to achieve a certain level of professional growth, I will disgrace my institute. Needless to say, it is another issue I should work out with my analyst—my "eldest daughter complex"! Working on control cases is like in a Baby Crawling Contest: being an analyst-in-training, I am as clumsy as a baby. No matter how supervisors and sponsoring committee members try to show directions, offer instructions, and cheer you up, there are still a lot of distractions and obstacles on which you could easily stumble. The road is a bit bumpy, and luckily, I have reached my last mile to the endpoint.

Dear Institute, 30 years since I first read the mandarin translation of *Interpretation of Dreams*, I was finally accepted as a candidate. Am I a bit different now? I hope so. However, I also hope that the 18-year-old part of me still remains the same. I still remember how amazed I was when reading Freud, how curious I was when facing my patients, and how astonished I was when I got to know more of my own psychic world. Twenty years ago, I told my patient that I had to leave my job as a psychiatrist for some time because I wanted to study psychoanalysis in London. My patient, a university student with a philosophy major, asked me: "Why? Is psychoanalysis not out of date?" I am not sure if psychoanalysis is really out of date, or is it merely a diminished clinical practice, but I am sure it is a way of thinking and living. You look at things in different dimensions, and it changes me into a slightly different and, hopefully, better person. Better because I am more honest and more in touch with myself.

Taiwan Psychoanalytical Society is a new group waiting for future development. Our situation is very unique because we need to find a way to coordinate the Institute and Allied Center. I don't know how the fourth region of

IPA will develop in Asia, what I can contribute would be to participate in the psychoanalytic movement in Taiwan. Though we still have a long way to go, I can't wait to join you as analyst in the near future.

— Nancy Pei-Ling Yu

## Notes

1 Dr. Tsai later became the first president of Taiwan Center for the Development of Psychoanalysis.
2 Rudie Vermote, training analyst of the Belgian Society of Psychoanalysis; Michael Gundle, training analyst of the Seattle Psychoanalytic Society and Institute (SPSI). They are members of the Sponsoring Committee for Taiwan Study Group. According to the bylaws of IPA, local training by Taiwan Study Group is done with the help and supervision of its sponsoring committee. The first group of candidates of Taiwan Study Group were interviewed by Rudi and Michael.

# 39 Another letter to the Taiwan Center for the Development of Psychoanalysis, Taipei (2018)

*I-Ning Yeh*

*(Editor's note: For a brief history of the Taiwan Center for the Development of Psychoanalysis, please refer to the letter by Nancy Pei-Ling Yu.)*

*The training is in accordance with IPA regulations and following a modified Eitingon model. The training programs consist of three parts: personal analysis, four-year curriculum seminars, and case supervision. To be qualified as a psychoanalyst, candidates must be authorized by the Progression Committee, formed of the sponsoring committee as well as three training analysts in the Taiwan Study Group. Our personal analysis starts before training commences and continues through its course. Candidates also need to complete a four-year curriculum and continue attending clinical seminars until completion of the training. We are required to complete at least two control cases, each of which has to continue for at least two years, with a frequency of supervisory sessions of normally once a week for at least 40 supervisory sessions per year. Finally, we are required to do an oral presentation of our control cases to the Progression Committee. These requirements reinforce each other and provide a complete and multi-faceted learning experience.*

—

Dear Institute,

When I have been considering what I might say to you, my dear institute, a very young nurturer, so many thoughts, recollections, and reflections come to mind. I decided to allow myself to look retrospectively, to associate freely, to discover what has happened in my personal journey of studying psychoanalysis. I believe I am not the only, nor will I be the last, Asian who has struggled to find a way to study psychoanalysis, a subject developed in the West, and to continue my studies while maintaining my life and work in my own country. I hope that sharing my experiences will be of some values.

Dear Institute, when I was a 10-year-old girl, I read the Chinese translation of a psychology book I had found in the corner of the neighborhood library. I cannot remember the name of the book, but I remember it mentioned

DOI: 10.4324/9781003465409-39

something like "original-me (本我, id)", "self-me (自我, ego)" and "superior-me (超我, superego)". I was fascinated by the idea that there could be three kinds of me in myself, and that they could interact with each other. A couple of years later, I graduated from medical school and then started my training in a psychiatric residency. I was still interested in studying how the human mind works and believed that we can cure patients not only through chemical medication but also through words, or by helping patients gradually discover the truth about themselves.

To further my studies and learn about more advanced psychotherapeutic treatments, I went to University College London in 2005, attending the course of "Studies on Theoretical Psychoanalysis". I also started the seven-year journey to have psychoanalysis five times a week, including personal, online, and shuttle sessions. I remember in my first interview with my British analyst, telling him I was worried about the limitations of my ability to express myself through foreign language, as well as the great difference between our socio-cultural backgrounds. Dear institute, to my surprised, my very experienced British analyst told me, "Don't worry, the unconscious will find its way". And it did work! During the analysis, I found the childhood memories, dreams, and associations, like pieces of a jigsaw puzzle, fit together when we came to the realization of the lost parts of myself. I appreciated the help I got from my own analysis and considered becoming a psychoanalyst. I started doing more psychoanalytic therapies to help my patients, just as these therapies had helped me. However, at that time, there was no training institute in Taiwan, and I had to go abroad to seek further psychoanalytic training, which would take a couple of years. I was hesitant at first, and finally, because of family commitments and my own limited finances, I had no choice but to give up my dream, as painful as this was.

Dear Institute, I really appreciate all of the pioneer analysts of you and would like to let you know that I am so grateful to become one of the first eight candidates. I was initially hesitant about applying and wondered whether it would mean having to give up my full-time job. My out-patient hospital clinic work had its limitations, but it was helpful to the patients not able to afford either the time for, or the cost of, psychoanalysis, or even for psychotherapy. The dean of our hospital, a catholic sister, who could see beyond the need for the hospital to be able to turn a profit and she also understood and believed in the power of invisible mental connection between people. After I told her of my plans, she indulged me as much as she could in terms of my job during the training period. Dear institute, I live in southern Taiwan, so I would travel 400 km for my own analytic sessions in central Taiwan and 720 km for the training seminars in northern Taiwan. Although not inconsiderable, I found these distances acceptable, especially considering the fact that I would need to travel 9,800 km to get back to London. This distance was made even less formidable by the High-Speed Rail, without which attending the training course would have been far more difficult. Since 2018, I have traveled on the HSR three days a week to attend the analyses and training courses. I find the best way of dealing with all of the difficulties is just treating it as part of life and persisting with the training. At the end of the day, all the help and experience I have received has been beneficial to me, and I am still reaping the rewards of this psychoanalytic journey and the training I received.

Dear Institute, since March 2018, all the candidates have been meeting every Saturday afternoon on the 19th floor of a building over a metro station in central Taipei. Looking out from the big windows of the top of the building, we enjoyed the splendid views outside while reading and discussing psychoanalytic materials broadening our inner perspectives. We shared handmade bread and cookies, fresh fruit and cakes as we shared our clinical findings, week after week. It was hugely beneficial to be able to join my work with the patients, my own analysis and psychoanalytic papers together within the dynamic of the discussion. The experience has been so inspiring, and the candidates work so well together, and I am fully confident that our friendship will continue even after we have finished our training.

The emerging tradition of developing psychoanalysis in Taiwan, which has been called the "Formosa Model" (Liu, 2013)[1] Our teacher analysts come from different training associations and societies around the world, including from Boston, Seattle, New York, London, and Paris. This "pluralistic" institute is open to different points of view. Through the selection of the essential psychoanalytical papers and the discussion of the clinical seminars, the candidates are given the opportunity to experience the diverse theoretical and clinical approaches of our teachers. They may emphasize different analytic perspectives or prefer different theories, depending on their own individual backgrounds, but even when not in full agreement with each other, they still respect each other and continue talking and discussing the items during the monthly study group meetings. The supervising analysts receive our feedback and suggestions every semester. I personally feel that I am shown respect and am being listened to during the training process. The study group members express their thoughts and try to understand the dynamics of the meetings, and there is an understanding that the rules can be changed if they are no longer felt to be relevant. After all, the teachers and candidates have evolved together over the course of this initial training program.

Dear Institute, in the approach of our teachers running the study group, I get a real sense of the spirit of the concept of "containing diversity and bridging differences", which also happened to be the theme of the IPA 4th Asia Pacific Conference, which was held in January 2023 in India. Despite inherent differences in approach, they nevertheless find ways to keep communication open and to maintain connections. During my time studying in the group, I learned that there are no such things as "correct" psychoanalytic concepts, just different psychoanalytic approaches to diverse mental processes. I learned to remain open to uncertainties and to exercise patience in the psychoanalytic listening. Although it took some time to arrive at this realization, it has proven very helpful to be flexible in terms of perspectives and even techniques in our clinical practices.

Dear Institute, I have realized that having my personal analysis was the best decision I have ever made. I am convinced of the timelessness and limitlessness of the unconscious because the interpretations and associations of my first analysis, which had finished many years ago, reappeared from time to time in my second analysis. My Taiwanese analyst is excellent, and very experienced. She has helped me see my defenses at the same time as realizing the reasons for them and finally being able to accept them as parts of myself. With her patience and assistance in the face of some very challenging analytic moments, the forgotten memories and unsolved mysteries gradually reappeared before me. I believe my analyst is a beacon of light, guiding me forward. She won't give me the answers directly but lit up the way before me. Not until I was lying on the couch again did I realize how much I love and have missed psychoanalysis. I was excited and sometimes scared because I would never know at the beginning of the session where I would end up. I feel the coach is like a space capsule, transporting me through the universe of the mind, allowing me to reach unknown destinations just by lying down. What kind of other travel is comparable to this?

Dear Institute, when I first tried to find patients willing to undergo intensive treatment, the response I got was generally doubt about how it could ever work. It is not so easy to convince our patients, even our psychiatrist colleagues, to accept psychoanalytic treatment, owing in great part, I believe, to Eastern culture, in which people are too embarrassed to talk about the "skeletons in their closets". People tend not to tell outsiders, including psychotherapists, their painful secrets and traumas related to their families and early life experiences. Fortunately, I do have some very courageous patients who were willing to open their minds and to work with me analytically with intensive sessions. I can see the psychic changes they have gone through when they gradually improve their relationships, first with themselves and then with others, and finally change their lives and fates: it is an amazing job to do. Although I learned from my own experiences and from my supervisors that psychoanalysis is not a perfect method that can solve each and every problem or be suitable for everyone, I am sure this is the best way to help my patients, for it helps us to think and look within, regardless of the circumstances.

Dear Institute, the training is coming to an end, but I know that my relationship with psychoanalysis and with you will continue. Looking back over the last decade, I know that the 2012-me would be so surprised how far I have come and how close I am to realizing my dream. I think that is the reason I would like to write to you, to express my appreciation for the help from you, my dear institute. The only word I can think of that adequately expresses how I feel about what I have experienced in my own personal analyses and the seminars, supervisions, and the work with my patients, is "love". Love creates connections. None of this would have been possible without you, my dear institute. I really appreciate the administrative work, the company, and the teaching I received during the training. I want to repay you by trying my best to pass the love from you to this new generation and the next. I will keep psychoanalysis alive and blossoming in Taiwan and pass it to our future candidates.

With best wishes,

— I-Ning Yeh

## Note

1 Taiwan has been long known as Formosa, which means "Beautiful Island". During the past few centuries, Taiwan has been governed by several different sovereign-ties. The blending of different languages, cultures, and customs in Taiwan gives rise to the richness and diversities in our society. "The Formosa Model" represents the developing psychoanalysis in Taiwan, "taking the diversity more as a strength than a flaw, we have encouraged our members to take an openminded and respectful attitude to different (psychoanalytic) schools".

# 40 A letter to Asociación Panameña de Psicoanálisis, Panama City (2020)

## Hildegarde Kochman

*Requirements for graduation:*

1. *Training analysis of three times a week with an additional session (duration convened between analyst and analysand) until control cases are completed.*
2. *Four years of seminars: theory, technique, clinical supervision.*
3. *Two control cases of three sessions weekly each: 100 hours of supervision per case, meetings once a week per case until completion of 100 hours plus written reports every 50 and 100 hours.*

*Historical information provided by Dr. Samuel Pinzón, Panamanian training analyst from Panamanian Psychoanalytic Society (APAP):*

*The precursor of APAP was a psychotherapy institute founded in 1977. A later development began in 1989, with three women who brought to Panama an extension of the International Institute for Object Relations Training/International Psychotherapy Institute (IIORT/IPI) to provide clinical training. It was under the sponsorship of ILAP (Latin-American Institute of Psychoanalysis), soon after its creation in 2007, that five Panamanians started their psychoanalytical formal training to become analysts and later training analysts. Four other male analysts were confirmed as well, to become training analysts of the region, which paved the way for the local Allied Center of Panamá to become the Psychoanalytic Study Group of Panamá (GEPP) in 2014. The Panamanian Psychoanalytical Association (APAP) has conquered the IPA membership level of a provisional society since January 2020 through the Liaison Committee, which brings new societies to gain full membership. Four Venezuelan psychoanalysts became part of the Institute, contributing with their experience and dedication to the training of new aspiring analysts. Eight of the 11 psychoanalysts at the Institute are training analysts today. Two groups of analysts-in-training who started in 2015 and 2019, respectively, have finished seminars, and four analysts have completed all training requirements.*

—

DOI: 10.4324/9781003465409-40

Dear Institute:

In one of many spontaneous conversations with other attendees during the IPA Congress in London in 2019, one analyst-in-training from a South American country shared her discomfort about what she called "being treated like a child" during her training. This concern made me wonder whether this was a common feeling among analysts-in-training since I had entertained the thought myself. Reviewing some experiences around this topic, makes me think that these feelings could be the result of initiating a journey that requires a certain amount of regression to a place of dependence, loss of autonomy, and not knowing.

One of the most difficult things about training is that we are already professionals in the field of mental health, but we are training for advancement in a new science called psychoanalysis. And we do need a lot of guidance as we enter a new realm of knowledge that will influence our work as clinicians. Accepting the challenge to start training requires us to become followers of psychoanalysis. And as disciples, we accept the notion of being led somewhat blindly. So that is one area in which ambivalence plays out.

As analysts-in-training, we need to learn from those who have been there before us as well as resign to a degree of autonomy since we enroll in a program that requires us to follow institutional rules with little space for dissent. One of those rules is committing to a training analysis which is not only necessary to learn the trade; we also have a place to grieve when feeling the regressive pulls from the infantile in our unconscious. With this I am implying everything that could become an obstacle in our training as well as our analysis. Having been in analysis for one year before my initiation of the training, and later turning it into a training analysis may have built a certain pressure as an analysand, something that I had not contemplated. I remained with the same analyst who also had other positions given the nature of our small institute. I now wonder how much of the regulations to "protect" the candidates, are effective on a selective basis. After several years of analysis, I opted for changing analysts, a decision that perhaps should have been taken before, if I had dared to think this through without fear of retaliation. In the meantime, all the pressures from the analysis and training made me oscillate between frustration and discontent, to wholesomeness and self-reliance striving to sustain myself both internally, by holding on to the capacity to withstand the strains of the program, as well as externally, by managing finances, day to day responsibilities and family time. We are making such an enormous effort; it just seems like the wish to be contained is not too much to ask. Not like a child, but as a human being committed to moving forward and fulfilling an aspiration.

In this pursuit to become psychoanalysts, we need analysts in our institutes to teach, hold, invest, and mentor. During my personal analysis, I once said that our institute should bring a parenting function into our development as psychoanalysts. So, you see, I admit that what is rejected is also what on occasion has been wished for. It wasn't quite this way that I articulated it, but I was describing hoping for more support and holding from the "elders". The way I pictured it was through an image of concentric circles, whereby as trainees, we stand on the inside surrounded (embraced) by this group of experienced psychoanalysts (who hold and support us) while overseeing and stimulating our growth.

That as advanced candidates and even not so advanced, we would be encouraged to participate in activities inside or outside our institute beyond required seminars. This longing to have been benefitted with a holding space from our teaching analysts perhaps is the maternal function that is necessary during times of endurance. This reminds me of the phrase "it takes a village to raise a child". This is such a warm concept about community, vulnerability, and bonds. And circles are figures of containment which define limits, but not to exclude but to include.

My thinking is that if we are not given the possibilities (the mentoring), then how would we mature our psychoanalytical abilities outside of the classroom and the consulting room? This I can say, as I have had a few opportunities to do this, but only because of my will and determination and by moving outside of my institute and finding other groups and mentors. In my fantasy, candidates would be allowed to participate in psychoanalytically oriented activities situated on the inside of this ideal circle I have created in my mind, held, and encouraged, but instead, I felt left on the outside, because of boundaries marked as to keep candidates in what I consider a subordinate position.

One time I was allowed to present an analysis of a film side by side with an analyst from my institute, whereby other candidates had had their turn before me, but suddenly, this modality was discontinued without an explanation. Later, we were encouraged to coordinate online activities with a visitor psychoanalyst which I did, but after much work, there was a sense of not getting full support as no one advised me of another important online meeting taking place on the same day. This, I recall, was a very frustrating experience, with mixed messages, but ultimately, not being taken seriously.

These activities continue to be promoted with the purpose of letting us have more participation within the institute, which makes me think that there is the will, but mine was an experience of a different sort. Dear institute, even in a psychoanalytical institution, analysts can sometimes make careless, insensitive mistakes.

Recently, I participated in a group discussion (mostly psychoanalysts) around this topic, whether analysts-in-training should be allowed to join and share spaces with psychoanalysts, and there was a 50/50 division of opinion for and against it. It dawned on me that the reason for not encouraging such interchange boils down to a transference issue and protecting the candidate's analysis. Can this essential element be challenged? If this is the case, we should be encouraged early on to practice exogamy and look for opportunities in other institutes and groups, especially now that there is virtual learning.

Also, what if, dear institute, not all training analysts are truly invested in their students' independence? Undoubtedly, as candidates, we want to feel we are maturing our psychoanalytical identities and abilities, something like what happens to adolescents (using the life cycle metaphor) who already have become resourceful in many ways, but who are dependent, not quite ready to separate, but in the process of consolidating a sense of self. When institutes are themselves young, going through their own growing pains, this may be an added burden to candidates who are receiving training but get caught up in the internal (dis)organization and bureaucracy involved in becoming an institute.

Having been trained in psychology and family therapy, and entering psychoanalysis with a great desire, I nevertheless, had little previous knowledge of metapsychology. This could be where my deep difficulties arose. Acceptance into our institute was contingent on having had one year of analysis, but our background was not an impediment. But never having studied Freudian theory was very straining. Despite this, I continued my training with eagerness. By the third year of seminars, I accepted the recommendation to receive tutoring. And this tutor also helped me put together my first collective presentation under the auspice of a committee. As it turned out, the need for tutoring became a blessing in disguise. The presentation mentioned above also proved a most valuable experience as researching deep into the subject of the "infantile" was of intrinsic value in my training. Writing essays and presentations gave us such opportunities that opened us to the discovery of new authors and areas of psychoanalysis we may want to pursue.

What I think I mean when I speak about the way I felt my institute failed me (and I realize I am using projection here) is that our professors should think about us as "grown-up children" who are mature enough in some respects but not others. Isn't that what psychoanalysis avails and restores in us? So, there is ambivalence about returning to dependency and accepting not knowing while our training analysis is procuring in us the capacity to re-parent ourselves through a revision of how this process became installed and by using our analysts and training professors as objects. However, the confidence needed to improve our emotional assets as individuals and clinicians will hardly sprout from being handled as incapable or immature. Furthermore, there is a contradiction between treating us as children and expecting us to be independently minded and believing in ourselves to create, initiate, and abandon inhibitions.

So, going back to the training function of our institutes, I would say to professors that it is more important to be concerned about understanding our individual characteristics as candidates when we are having some difficulties or want to be considered as grown-ups even when special needs appear. In contrast, the similarity with a family group comes to mind again when I am reminded of a comment directed to me coming from one of the "parents", which I interpreted as a call for provocation of siblings' rivalry. What would be the sense of pointing out that a "younger sibling" was doing something remarkable outside the institute if it was not to send the message, that others are ahead, and children who make their parents proud are the ones that are worth mentioning? This sounds very infantile, but I am also reminded that training in psychoanalysis makes us stronger in our ego to be able to face all "truths" and rehash comments that may carry a double message.

And dear institute, training in psychoanalysis is very harsh on our egos. But as candidates, we still choose to continue which proves that we submit to the rules but never stop wanting to achieve "true" adulthood, in the interest of our future and our patients.

It is impossible to have a flawless curriculum since candidates have different needs and backgrounds. We learn psychoanalytical theory, most likely Freudian theory, or Lacanian (in some South American institutes) and although there is no right way to teach metapsychology or Freudian theory, I would point out that our psychoanalytical thought process can acquire more depth if in our training we would hear discussions about the differences in authors' perspectives, and their approaches to theorizing, what makes them unique or different, and the strength in their theories. This I have gained after having finished required seminars and joining other study groups with whom I have acquired an appreciation of Freud's investigative method and theory building and integrating more authors into my repertoire. This additional effort has helped me improve my conceptual knowledge. Integrating psychoanalytical language and thinking is a task that takes years beyond our initial training. And indeed, getting a head start by having studied some metapsychology would have been useful. I have also considered that Freudian theory must be learned in chronological order and sometimes, less is more. His basic texts are full of proposals that if I had been able to study carefully in my early learning, perhaps, I would have done a better integration. Also, it is evident that the acquisition of such knowledge involves both primary and secondary processes.

Four years of seminars have come to an end, and there is relief from all the work that weighs heavily on our time and relationships. When arriving at this first goal of our training, the loss of the group meetings weekly and frequency of communications represented a new challenge, that of losing the containment of the training group. When the time comes, we all need to go our separate ways, but are we prepared to let go of colleagues at that moment? The bond created after significant hours spent together feels like a fraternity that, nevertheless, gets disbanded. On the one hand, I could hear some professors say that this is a natural and necessary process, while on the other, there was a contradiction in hearing we should join forces to continue learning. This separation can be difficult because the sharing has built such affectionate bonds; eventually, this gets sublimated with other study groups or by joining a committee or other areas in which to build new relationships. Dear institute, I felt unprepared for the end which left me with a sense of loss. The group represents a very intimate experience that even family and friends cannot empathize with. Psychoanalysis can have its lonely moments. But not everything is lost, some of us have continued meeting after the pandemic, and the internet is a good source for rekindling our relations and joining new study groups. Selection of control cases during training can be a hazardous area. As we moved along the training, our clinical professors prompted us to be ready to advance with our clinical patients. For anyone who hasn't seen patients more than once a week, this must be the most challenging aspect of the training. This can only be learned by trial and error unless the clinician is so experienced that this ability can be grasped by intuition and finesse. I learned the hard way that this ability would develop from the sum of my own developmental changes in my analysis, training seminars, and case supervisions. But this process is seldom discussed as such. I delayed my supervisions, for lack of clarity and fear of not being able to find a patient fitting into the category of analyzability. It was later that I realized why supervision itself is the springboard for entering patients into psychoanalytical treatments.

During those early years of training, it was suggested that patients would readily accept our proposal of coming three times weekly only because we proposed that the treatment called for it. I was told, that for patients to believe in psychoanalysis, we had to believe in psychoanalysis ourselves. I certainly struggled with that core concept of the construction of our psychoanalytical identity. Being able to read the patients' transference became an important tool to aim for someone that would fit into the profile of a potential psychoanalytical patient. And this, I had to learn, would be achieved through supervision of first-time patients. Waiting for the right patient seemed like an endless process whereby my own anxiousness could have gotten in the way as this would certainly appear in my countertransference. Supervision of patients who were not particularly adaptable to psychoanalytical treatment was demoralizing. Once control cases got in the way, I stopped feeling persecuted.

These are all aspects of becoming analysts that could be expressed in a more didactic way, although I also realize this type of knowledge will be integrated as part of the process of acquiring this psychoanalytical identity I have already mentioned.

Another misconception was that we would analyze neurotic patients. Only after failing with my first control case did I understand that this patient was more borderline than neurotic and that this type of personality disorder has a different modality of treatment. I have also learned that our training supervisors tend to be aligned with certain theories that may not fit every patient. Becoming more cautious in the treatment of these patients that are not the standard neurotic patient that I was trained during seminars to encounter, has been part of the necessary, but painful process. I supervise as much as I can, not just control cases. I join group supervisions and study other authors that teach us how to approach and diagnose patients whose personality falls within borderline states. Although these patients are more difficult to treat and to hold on to, as analysts-in-training, we become much more attuned to their suffering.

So, I conclude that there is no right way to teach and learn psychoanalysis. There were areas in my training that could be improved, but there is nothing so far that I have not been able to overcome in the practice. I tend to be a critic, but I would do it all over again.

By taking responsibility for several of my own missteps, and accepting what cannot be changed, I have become a humbler person and clinician, assets that surely, I take away from having had this training. And certainly, as candidates we agree to release some autonomy and to conform to institutional rules and regulations. Nonetheless, we must take chances occasionally, even when dissenting would be a departure from expected behavior.

No one escapes going through trials and tribulations when it comes to pursuing an idea(l), a desire, or knowledge. When I embarked on this journey, called psychoanalytic training, I had no idea of the effort that it would involve hoping to reach my destination (destiny). It has been long, winding, slippery, but also exciting, fulfilling, generative, and much more. I keep reminding myself that I must continue to enjoy the journey, but will I miss the roads traveled once I finish this training?

— Hildegarde Kochman
Analyst-in-training

# References

AIT Orientation Manual Committee. (2023). *AIT orientation manual* (p. 5). Western Canada Psychoanalytic Institute.

Agrawal, H. (2022, Winter). Trials and tribulations of being a candidate. *The American Psychoanalyst*.

Aslan, C. (1980). La experiencia argentina I. *Revista de Psicoanálisis, 37*(1), 147–158.

Baranger, M. (2003). Formación psicoanalítica, la reforma del '74, 30 años después. *Revista de la Asociación Psicoanalítica Argentina, 6*(4), 1043–1050.

Benjamin, W. (2003). On some motifs in Baudelaire. In E. Jephcott, H. Eiland, & M. W. Jennings (Eds.), *Walter Benjamin: Selected writings, Vol. 4, 1938–1940* (pp. 315–355). Belknapp Press-an imprint of Harvard University Press. (Original work published 1940)

Bion, W. R. (1984). Differentiation of the psychotic from the non-psychotic personalities. In *Second thoughts* (pp. 43–65). Karnac Books. (Original work published 1957)

Bion, W. R. (2014). Two papers: The grid and caesura. In C. Mawson (Ed.), *The complete works of W. R. Bion* (Vol. 10). Taylor & Francis. (Original work published 1977)

Bissonnette, N. (2022, March). Freud et nous. *Bulletin de la société psychanalytique de Montréal, 34*(1).

Blass, R. B. (2010). How does psychoanalytic practice differ from psychotherapy? The implications of the difference for the development of psychoanalytic training and practice: "An introduction to distinguishing psychoanalysis from psychotherapy". *The International Journal of Psychoanalysis, 91*(1), 15–21.

Bolognini, S. (2008). A família institucional e a fantasmática do analista. *Jornal de Psicanálise, 41*(74).

Bolognini, S. (2014, May). *Hacia un modelo cuatripartito: "Towards a quadripartite model"*. International Psychoanalytical Association. Newsletter to the Members.

Boots, J. (2010, January). What to do about Australia. *Psychoanalysis Downunder, 10*.

Busch, F. (2020). *Dear candidate: Analysts from around the world offer personal reflections on psychoanalytic training, education, and the profession*. Routledge.

Caldwell, L., & Joyce, A. (2011). *Reading Winnicott*. Taylor & Francis.

Calich, J. C., Hartke, R., Levy, R., & Lewkowicz, S. (1995, November). A idealização e seus desvios na formação analítica: Novas reflexões. *Revista de Psicanálise da SPPA, II*(3), 455–463.

Carlino, R. (2010). *Psicoanálisis a distancia*. Lumen.

Carroll, L. (2000). *Alice's adventures in wonderland*. Broadview Press.

Chessman, H., & Wayt, L. (2016). What are students demanding? *Higher Education Today*.

Dickinson, E. (1998). *The poems of Emily Dickinson: Reading edition*. The Belknap Press of Harvard University Press.

Di Lampedusa, G. T. (1958). *The leopard*. Vintage.

Eaton, J. (2015). Building a floor for experience: A model for thinking about children's experience. In N. Tracey (Ed.), *Transgenerational trauma and the aboriginal preschool child, healing through intervention* (pp. 43–70). Rowman & Littlefield.

Ehrlich, L. T. (2012). The analyst's reluctance to begin a new analysis. In *Initiating psychoanalysis: Perspectives*. Routledge.

Freud, S. (1964). The question of lay analysis: Conversation with an impartial person. In *An autobiographical study: Inhibitions, symptoms and anxiety* (pp. 177–258). Hogarth, The Institute of Psychoanalysis. (Original work published 1926)

Freud, A. (1968). The evaluation of applicants for psychoanalytic training. *International Journal of Psychoanalysis, 49*, 548–554.

Freud, S. (1993). El creador literario y el fantaseo. En J. L. Etcheverry (Traduc), *Obras Completas: Sigmund Freud* (Vol. 9, pp. 123–135). Buenos Aires. Amorrortu (Trabajo original publicado en 1908)

Furlong, A. (2020). *Dear candidate* (F. Busch, Ed., pp. 73–75). Routledge.

García, J. (2011). The training of psychoanalysts in Latin American countries without IPA institutions: Antecedents, experiences and problems encountered. *The International Journal of Psychoanalysis, 92*(3), 715–731. https://doi.org/10.1111/j.1745-8315.2011.00464.x

Jackson, P. W. (1968). *Life in classrooms*. Holt, Rinehart and Winston, Inc.

Jacobs, T. J. (1994). Nonverbal communications: Some reflections on their role in the psychoanalytic process and psychoanalytic education. *Journal of the American Psychoanalytic Association, 42*, 741–762.

Kellman, J., & Radwan, K. (2022). Towards an expanded neuroscientific understanding of social play. *Neuroscience & Biobehavioral Reviews, 132*, 884–891.

Kernberg, O. F. (1996). Thirty methods to destroy the creativity of psychoanalytic candidates. *International Journal of Psychoanalysis, 77*, 1031–1040.

Klein, M. (1989). *The psycho-analysis of children*. Virago. (Original work published 1932)

Kolke, R. (2022, August). *Seminar on self psychology*. Israel Psychoanalytic Society.

Lacan, J. (2006). The mirror stage as formative if the I function as revealed in psychoanalytic experience. In B. Fink (Trans.), *Ecrits: The first complete edition in English*. W. W. Norton and Company. (Original work published 1949)

Laplanche, J. (1992). Transference: Its provocation by the analyst. In *Reading French psychoanalysis*. Routledge.

Leeds, A. M. (2009). *A guide to the standard EMDR protocols for clinicians, supervisors, and consultants* (pp. 71–72). Springer Publishing Company.

Liu, C. C. (2013). The Formosa model: An emerging tradition of developing psychoanalysis in Taiwan. In A. Gerlach (Ed.), *Psychoanalysis in Asia* (pp. 225–236). Karnac Books.

Logan, J. (1958). *South Pacific* [Film]. South Pacific Enterprises.

Makari, G. (2009). *Revolution in mind: The creation of psychoanalysis*. Harper Perennial.

Marion, P. (2022). *The transmission of psychoanalysis: An ideal object and its risks*. EPF-Congress.

McCartney, P. (1967). *With a little help from my friends*. Sgt. Pepper's Lonely Hearts Club Band. Parolphone-Capitol records.

O'Connor, K. (2003). *The history of the Baltic states*. Greenwood Press.

Panksepp, J. (1998). *Affective neuroscience: The foundations of human and animal emotions*. Oxford University Press.

Quinodoz, J. (2004). *Lire Freud*. PUF.

Roussillon, R. (2018). *Manuel de psychologie et de psychopathologie clinique générale*. Elsevier Masson.

Solms, M. (2021a). *The hidden Spring: A journey to the source of consciousness.* Profile Books Limited.

Solms, M. (2021b). A revision of Freud's theory of the biological origin of the Oedipus complex. *The Psychoanalytic Quarterly, 90*(4), 555–581.

Sousa, N. C. (2021, February 7). *Wilfred Bion, Tavistock clinic seminars— August 4, 1978* [Video]. YouTube. Retrieved September 26, 2022, from https://www.youtube.com/watch?v=kuE_JepuqDw

St. Amour, M. (2020). As times and students change, can faculty change too? *Inside Higher Ed.*

Tomasel, E. (2016). Um balanço entre as ondas do passado e as atuais: reflexões sobre a fase inicial de formação psicanalítica. *Revista de Psicanálise da Sociedade Psicanalítica de Porto Alegre, 23*(3), 559–567.

Volkan, V. D. (2013). *Enemies on the couch: A psychopolitical journey through war and peace.* Pitchstone Publishing.

Vygotsky, L. S. (1978). *Mind in society: Development of higher psychological processes.* Harvard University Press.

Winnicott, D. W. (1960). The theory of the parent-child relationship. *International Journal of Psychoanalysis, 41*, 585–595.

Winnicott, D. W. (1971a). Creativity and its origins. In *Playing and reality* (pp. 65–85). Brunner Routledge (1991).

Winnicott, D. W. (1971b). Mirror-role of mother and family in child development. In *Playing and reality* (pp. 111–118). Brunner Routledge (1991).

Winnicott, D. W. (1971c). *Cap 1 Objetos transicionales y fenómenos transicionales de "Realidad y juego"* (pp. 17–45). Gedisa Editorial.

Winnicott, D. W. (2017a). Creativity and its origins. In L. Caldwell & H. Taylor Robinson (Eds.), *The collected works of D. W. Winnicott* (Vol. 9). Taylor & Francis. (Original work published 1971)

Winnicott, D. W. (2017b). Playing: Creative activity and the search for the self. In L. Caldwell & H. Taylor Robinson (Eds.), *The collected works of D. W. Winnicott* (Vol. 8). Taylor & Francis. (Original work published 1971)

Winnicott, D. W. (2017c). Transitional objects and transitional phenomena. In L. Caldwell & H. Taylor Robinson (Eds.), *The collected works of D. W. Winnicott* (Vol. 9). Taylor & Francis. (Original work published 1971)

Woodall, T., Hiller, A., & Resnick, S. (2012). Making sense of higher education: Students as consumers & the value of the university experience. *Studies in Higher Education, 39*(1).

Zac de Filc, S. (2002). Psicoanálisis y futuro. *Revista de Psicoanálisis, 59*(2), 329–341.

# Index